Care giving a loved one is such ɛ
read for those who are currently (
Marriage, Family, therapist, I also
understand what many of th̲ ̲ ̲ ̲ ̲ ̲ ̲ ̲ ̲ ̲ ̲ ̲ ̲ ̲ experiencing.

Marie Derrick
Retired Marriage and Family Therapist

I have been a part time care giver for both my mother and father as well as a full
time care giver for a spouse through the entire Alzheimer's process.

I find this book has a great many useful suggestions and tips for care givers in
almost any situation. It would also be very helpful to the care giver to know that
he / she is not alone in the process, and that there are some options for help.

Tom Fisher
Seattle, WA

My husband was ill for several years and it became my responsibility not only to
care of his physical needs but to take over the responsibilities of all our family,
financial and emotional needs. To have such a resource available as Durlynn
Anema's book on care giving would not only have been helpful to me, but would
have given some peace of mind to my husband to know there was help available I
could use to ease my burden. It was a three year struggle and it would have been
so much easier, especially during the last year to learn ways to cope with my
husband as well as myself.

Elma Griffin
Astoria, OR

In a six month period of time I lost a fifty-six year-old brother to a quick battle
with liver cancer, and two grandmothers to the slow process of age {one was
ninety-eight, and the other ninety-nine). In neither case was I prepared, nor knew
what to do. I could have used Durlynn's book on love and duty in processing the
time of care for these precious family members, the medical mazes of seeming
incompetence, and difficult decisions that caused such pain and disagreements
in both sides of my family. It is always easier to follow someone who has walked
in those situations.

Karen D. Wood, Licensed Clinical Social Worker, Author *of Brain Prayers:
Explore Your Brain, Expand Your Prayers*

Elma –

Thank you for your comments about the relevance of my book. You always show strength and faith – a great example for others.

Durlynn Anema

LOVE OR DUTY?

A JOURNEY IN CAREGIVING

BY

DURLYNN ANEMA, PH. D. AND
FAMILY COUNSELOR

ISBN 13: 978-0-88100-160-0
ISBN10: 0-88100-160-0
Library of Congress Number: 2014908123

Cover Design by NZ Graphics

Published by National Writers Press, Inc. ™

Library of Congress Cataloging-in-Publication Data

Anema, Durlynn
Love or Duty?: A Journey in Caregiving by Durlynn Anema, Ph. D.

International Standard Book Number 13: 978-0-88100-160-0
International Standard Book Number 10: 0-88100-160-0

1. Family & Relationships/ General   2. Family & Relationships / Eldercare
3. Family & Relationships / Education   I. Title   2014908123

Dedicated to my husband Vern who now is on his newest journey -- and to all caregivers who must experience this journey in their own ways.

TABLE OF CONTENTS

A JOURNEY

You're about to take a journey in care giving -- meeting people directly involved in a rapidly growing event in our aging society. It's a journey with highs and lows, joys and frustrations, smiles and anger. It may well be yours -- either as the caregiver or the one being cared for.

Essentially, there are two types of care giving -- for older adults and for developmentally disabled and handicapped children. Your journey focuses on caring for the older adult.

You're going to meet fantastic people who care and nurture from the bottom of their souls. Realistic people who care because they've been thrust into a new life. And people who wonder and still can't believe they're in this position.

Much of the journey will be seen from my perspective because I was a 24/7 care giver for three plus years. You'll also hear the stories of many other men and women --most of whom were thrust into a role they never envisioned happening. Scattered throughout are the professionals who come into caregiving because it's part of their nurturing personalities.

Come along on this journey -- experience the lives of people I met from all corners of the U. S. -- and know this is a special journey that is done with both LOVE AND DUTY.

PREFACE

You never suspected it would happen to you -- until now. You might be a spouse, a child of the older adult, a family member, or a close friend. Whatever your status, you have a new role -- one we take on because we love the individual or feel a duty to perform all tasks, no matter the consequences.

A new role!! One interviewee strongly emphasized, not once but several times, that there are no "one size fits all" cases in caregiving. Each caregiver is faced with circumstances different from anyone else. So hopefully, any crumb from interviews will help you through this difficult time.

And don't kid yourself -- this time will be a difficult one as you try to do the very best for the person you love. Bright days occur when everything goes great -- when your loved one is cheery and aware of his or her surroundings. Frustrating days occur when everything goes wrong -- from your inability to satisfy your loved one to the messes you have to clean. You can get through all incidents if you tell yourself you are doing the best you can.

You may be involved in one of three types of caregiving. Caregiving 1 is that of spouse or older parent (and combinations thereof) in which you'll care for that person in your home. Be aware at some point this becomes a 24/7 job -- or as one interviewee said "And many hours added to that!" You may not be getting much sleep, may be on the alert at all times for the wandering spouse/parent or the accidents that "weren't meant to happen." This is a burden, no matter how you say it, especially if you are the only one involved in the caregiving -- if there aren't relatives or close friends who can occasionally relieve you. This is Caregiving 1.

Caregiving 2 is the loved one who has become so incapacitated he or she must be placed in a skilled nursing (or similar) facility because you cannot care for the person in your home for any number of reasons (small home, work, number of children, etcetera). You may hear the comment, "Oh that person is in a nursing home so we don't have to worry about them." This is far from the case. If you really love that person, you will organize your schedule to include that person in your day or as close to every day as you can. Nursing home environments range from excellent to so poor you wouldn't want your loved one there. But even the finest facilities need your constant attention, as does your loved one. You can't visit at the same time every day -- going for different meal times, at morning or afternoon when your loved one is up, or in the evening to watch those procedures. Nursing home personnel will recognize your schedule -- and that you care. This gives them incentive to care, also.

Finally, comes Caregiving 3 where your loved one still is in his or her own home but needs your constant attention (actually relies on that attention). While they can do simple tasks for themselves like getting easy meals and doing light cleaning, they still need watching. You never know when they might fall or have a problem in the bath. You have to be prepared to call the home bound person each day. If your loved one doesn't answer, you must go to his or her home or have an emergency person check. Probably, your loved one no longer can drive (or shouldn't!), so you'll have to arrange your schedule to take them to doctor's appointments, or to the grocery store. Naturally, this person can't stay in his or her home 24/7, so you'll have to plan lunch dates and times with you and your family at your house. Obviously, this caregiving experience isn't any less time consuming.

All three types of caregiving will be covered because I am in the unique role of having experienced all three -- with my mother in her own apartment, with my grandmother in a skilled nursing facility, with my husband in our home. My only difference with the first two was I was in my late twenties/early thirties while my spouse's care was while I was in my early seventies. But no matter the age -- and the energy component -- caregiving is a task.

May you find what you need through my and other people's experiences -- and know you are never alone.

WHY THIS TITLE?

Two weeks after Vern died my publisher suggested I write this book. She had watched my reactions as I cared for him and his progressive illness over the three and a half year period. She also knew how people often were amazed at my usual cheeriness, greeting them with a smile. Many people never sensed my true circumstances.

As I began to write the book, I realized it was an examination of many details often overlooked when discussing a caregiver role. I realized when any of us begin care of a loved one, the person is exactly that -- "a loved one," meaning we truly love that person. We want to help, so understand caregiving is now an integral part of our total life.

Caregiving happened to me several times in my life -- although never the 24/7 role I experienced with Vern, my husband. During all these circumstances, I knew I had been given a situation to perform and whether through love or duty, I performed it. However, as the months and even years passed that word "duty" crept into my vocabulary. Most of you won't want to admit that -- but caregiving is a duty that we know has to be performed each day.

This reality becomes clear when our loved one moves on from this life to another. I was talking to a woman who cared for her Alzheimer stricken mother for years. She sheepishly told me she felt such relief when her mother died -- then quickly added she didn't mean to say that.

Why not? Her life for many years was devoted to her mother's care -- just as my life was devoted to Vern's. When that finishes there has to be a sense of relief, even if we don't want to admit it.

It's not just relief for ourselves but also for the deceased person who has been through so much.

The title says it all. Most of us do love the person for whom we are caring. Yet, as the days slip by -- and the months and even years -- we wonder how much more we can undergo. We are frustrated -- and let's admit it, also angry -- because we wonder if it will ever end.

Then it does end. All those months and years are washed away -- like it was a small occurrence in our lives. I was surprised when I felt that way. Vern was gone and so were those days of wondering whether I would survive. Hence the title -- not in disrespect for the lost one, but in the sense that another phase of life is passed -- for both of us.

Outline of the Book

The chapters have been divided into areas with which you might relate. All chapters also have caregiver narrative examples of what others have faced. Chapter One, The Journey Begins, talks about my first reactions to what was happening to my husband. Chapter Two, Learning Facts about the Journey, encapsulates the many books and internet resources along with facts about caregiving.

Chapter Three, The Journey's Many Byways, looks at the many ways to care for older parents/grandparents and spouses. Then Parent/Child. Child/Parent Journey, Chapter Four, examines how the parent/child role changes as people age.

Chapter Five, Overcoming the Journey's Roadblocks, states the honest evaluation that this caregiving journey will not be easy. Then Chapter Six, A Journey to Age Related Dementia OR?, takes on the problem of Alzheimer's, the stages and ways to deal with it.

Chapters Seven and Eight talk about how to handle the journey --Chapter Seven's title is Shoulda/Coulda Aids for the Journey and Chapter Eight's is Never Stopping the Journey through car trips or other adventures.

Our Journey Ends -- Out of the Darkness is the final Chapter Nine. It talks about letting go and still loving.

CHAPTER ONE

THE JOURNEY BEGINS

Three years and three months -- that was the comment I was making a few months before my husband's death. I had worn down physically, mentally, and emotionally, and knew my patience was short. He felt it and began to say, "You'd be better off if I'd die."

Immediately, I countered with, "Of course not. We're okay. I'm just a little tired." But I knew how tired I really was. I'd lost almost fifteen pounds. I wasn't sleeping well, and realized I yelled more than I should. That attitude made me feel all the worse -- until I began to pray, "When will this end?"

Those aren't pleasant words, but at some time during this process you'll have to admit you also may say them. If you don't say them, then you are a saint -- and that's a title I'd never give myself.

Vern was diagnosed with COPD in 1998, over ten years before his death. He readily admitted it was his fault, that he had smoked since he was twelve. He grew up when smoking was encouraged, the "chic" way of living the sophisticated life. All the smart people smoked -- especially in the movies!

The scenario with COPD is a steady downhill spiral -- hard to walk long distances, breathing becoming more difficult, etc. By 2003, I wondered if we should take a cruise around Cape Horn because of his breathing problems. However, we continued to make the trips, buy a small place in the Palm Springs area (an inexpensive park model in an RV park), and move our fifth wheel to a place we could visit year around. By 2006, he wasn't playing golf any more -- it was too strenuous for him. And his time in the swimming pool was simply walking around (something he could do until the end).

In November 2007, he took a serious fall that broke his right cheek bones and nose, but no other bones. For the rest of his life he fell often, but all that milk he drank as a boy and the rest of his life created very strong bones. He never broke anything more, but his downhill spiral had begun.

By this time, his driving skills were impaired and he was starting to lose his eyesight. I had promised a trip to Branson, and decided driving would be better than flying. We went to Branson in May 2008, then to Mt. Rushmore, a total of almost five thousand miles -- all of which I drove. During the trip, he was having a hard time getting around. Consequently, I had to let him out at the theater, restaurant and lodging entrances, and always carry everything which had to be moved.

His strength continued to decrease. It was harder for him to walk down steps. I was always frightened when he got into our pool because it did not have a railing to hold on to. His eye sight continued to deteriorate. He was walking less and less and breathing harder. I tried another trip in July 2009 to Yellowstone, and realized this was the last big trip we could do. He sat in the car -- not even attempting to see things outside. We could no longer go to my daughter's home in Washington state because it was split level and I was worried about him falling down stairs. However, we still enjoyed ourselves, and at that juncture I didn't think about my increased workload.

The journey of caregiving is a steady progression -- unfortunately downward. Thankfully, there are the good days -- the ones we have to remember every minute of the journey. We also have to remember we are not the only ones going through this.

Caregiving has been an integral part of human lives throughout mankind's history. In the past, families cared for everyone in a household, young and old, because everyone lived together -- rich and poor. The normal caregiver was a woman -- which was expected because caregiving of children and older household members was part of her household duties.

Some facts need to be considered in the above scenario. The life span was much shorter -- perhaps no more than forty years. Also, the older person was considered a wise soul -- venerated in many world cultures up to today. In those times, would anyone have thought that people would actively live until their seventies, into their eighties and beyond?

Yet, in the civilized world today it has happened. Seventy, eighty and even ninety year olds are as active as people in their fifties once were. Take a look at old movies, where someone in their fifties looked and acted old. Then go to a retirement village where "old" people swim, golf, and play tennis. I never could have pictured my grandmothers doing that.

But with all that longer life span come some sober statistics. A person may live longer but not necessarily in good health. The more common diseases yet to be cured include Parkinson's, diabetes, and kidney problems. And the most devastating disease for too many families is Alzheimer's.

An interesting observation about this new aging dynamic is that the caregiver role has changed. Yes, the major caregiver still is a woman, often in her late forties or fifties and caring either for a parent (sometimes grandparent) or a spouse. But a new person has been added -- the spouse of a woman with an acute illness or Alzheimer's. Men now are in the equation performing duties usually relegated to women.

Vern's first wife had been ill for several years and essentially he was the caregiver. While I did not know the extent of his caregiving until we met, I was aware of it by the way he wheeled her into and out of church and to their car. He told me the care became a 24/7 job toward the end of her life and he was thankful she was small and easy to carry. He also declared he never would have not taken care of her: they had been married over forty years.

At our place in the Palm Springs area, I noticed a couple who often were in the hot tub or at the pool at the same time as Vern and I. By that time, I was struggling to get Vern in and out of pools. I noticed the husband did virtually the same thing. When in the hot tub with that couple, Vern would talk almost incessantly and the wife would only smile when her husband answered. By the husband's actions -- taking her in and out of pools, being sure she hung on to a pool float, putting on her pool shoes -- I figured she had Alzheimers. (And learned later that the husband had been taking total care of her for almost six years.)

Consequently, both men and women now are caregivers, some the same ages as spouses, others younger, or children or grandchildren. Consequently, these caregivers find themselves leading completely different lives from their immediate past.

A Life Change

Caregiving changes lives -- both yours and that of the ill or older person. If the person for whom you are caring doesn't want anyone else to shower or dress him or her-- or take care of those very personal items -- what are you to do? This is when you recognize you are in a completely different life situation.

And one major thing about caregiving -- it is not a "one size fits all," as mentioned previously. I've read many caregiving books and none quite convey those moments when we wonder if we will survive. Many of you, male and female, are taking care of an ill spouse. Did we think our marriages would end in this drama of life? No, but we've accepted it as part of the words we said so very long ago -- "for better or for worse."

> *I'll never forget the beautiful note from one of Vern's sons-in-law. He wrote that he had gone to church one Sunday and heard a sermon on the seriousness of the marriage vows, "For better or worse."*
>
> *"It never dawned on me until I heard that sermon that you are now living the second part," he wrote. "And I'll think of you often now with what is happening to Vern AND to you."*

I cherished his words. This wasn't the first time I had been in a caregiving role. When taking care of my mother and my grandmother I was in my late twenties/early thirties. I probably had more energy at that time --evident by my duties to family, husband, and three young children!

My first caregiving roles were early in life, well before most of my peers. In today's society, many children in their forties, fifties, or sixties take care of a parent or parents -- or even a grandparent. Care may be in their homes, or through an assisted living or skilled nursing facility, or even with a parent living in his or her own home but needing help.

And never forget the parents who have been in caregiving roles for their children since the child's birth -- and will be in that role their entire life. I concentrate on elder caregiving because of the increasing number of older people. The fabulous parents and caregivers of disabled children deserve a huge salute in a separate book.

> *One interviewee said it well. "This is much more than a twenty-four hour job. It is several hours more each day. It is never completely sleeping. It is always being alert for whatever might happen."*
>
> *Another person said, "Caregiving does become duty at times. No matter how much we say we are doing everything out of love, there are times when we are tired or frustrated and yet have to go on -- the duty."*

Face it -- this is a time of change in your life. However, you learn when the ill person goes beyond to another life that the caregiving time washes away. Hopefully, then you will be left only with fond memories.

Nuances of Caregiving

Caregiving has many nuances, not just one dimension. Caregiving is such an exacting and all encompassing role that more than one time the caregiver feels totally overwhelmed. Don't be dismayed if you feel that way. You are only human and fragile -- and sometimes so tired you feel like giving up. While we have the love and duty to perform all tasks during the ill person's lifetime -- we also have to remember ourselves and what may be happening to us.

I want to convey in this book -- that while we have the love and duty to perform all tasks during the ill person's lifetime -- we also have to remember ourselves and what may be happening to us.

You'll look at what you need to do for yourselves in later chapters, but suffice it to say that you do need to think of yourselves in order to continue to care for your loved one. How many times have you seen the caregiver die before the "cared for" person? This especially seems to happen to men who seem so exhausted by their caregiving role that their body gives out. One man took on the care of his wife when she got Alzheimer's, then died of cancer while she still was alive.

You have to find an outlet for yourselves during that time -- even if it is simply sitting in front of the TV watching old movies. Think of something you can do in your home, if you don't have the luxury of a paid caregiver at least once a month -- painting, needlework, thinking up new recipes, gardening, reading, writing, or walking if you can slip away (very difficult with the Alzheimer's loved one). You need an activity to take your mind from your duties.

Try to maintain contact with the outside world. Vern's family lived quite a distance, and my sons and family were over thirty miles away. A few of our church family kept in touch after we stopped going to church -- but not many. If I met someone at the store and said, "Do come by" -- I rarely heard from them. Why? Quite often, it is difficult for people to see others in distress -- hard to visit an ill person. But those outside contacts help the housebound person and the caregiver. Don't stop trying to have these contacts.

As I look back, I should have realized what was happening to me and my mental attitude -- but I had so much to do I never knew what was actually happening to me. My saving grace during the three years and three months -- the two nonfiction books I wrote and the occasional client I saw for my counseling practice (which became almost nonexistent due to my husband's increasing illness).

If this sounds familiar to you (probably even saying, "Wait until she hears my story") it's because either you are experiencing it, or know someone who is. Caregivers who survive mentally and physically either have a deep faith, or have so much love in their hearts they accept whatever happens to them without question.

Mrs. "Y" thought her life now was perfect. She and her husband moved into their dream home on a golf course in their early sixties. Their children were a close thirty miles away so they could count on family time as well as time alone with each other -- something about which they always dreamed.

Then her husband had a severe stroke. After his rehabilitation, she brought him home. He could function -- could walk around, eat by himself and she could leave him alone -- but he never was able to sit and talk with her about what was happening in their lives or really enjoy the children and grandchildren.

Mrs. "Y" now was a 24/7 caregiver and would be for years. To date, he still is functioning and alive, able to dress himself and shower by himself but not able to participate with her in things they once did together. She has children close enough to relieve her of continuous duties -- and she found a volunteer job that takes her away from her home two to three mornings a week. These occurrences keep her sane as she ponders what will happen with the rest of her life.

My life changed, just as yours has or will change. I'm amazed at the circumstances I began to take as routine. When I had to get Vern in and out of a car it was just another task that had to be done (and he was quite heavy). Evidently, I gained strength because I always had to get him out of a chair and help him to his walker. And it didn't seem that hard.

He continued to fail. He hated the idea of a cane, never was able to function properly with one. A trip by a yard sale settled that problem when we found a walker for sale. He used this item for the rest of his life -- first simply when he was out of doors, and at the end all the time.

Life had become a new routine and I slipped so quickly into it that I hardly noticed all I was doing.

During Vern's first year with constricted movement we met an interesting couple at our Palm Springs place. We were all in the spa together when I noticed the husband kept up a good conversation with us while his wife simply smiled.

When the husband helped her out of the pool and then put on her shoes, we knew life was much more difficult for them. During the remainder of our time there I watched a husband devoted entirely to his wife and her problems.

The next year they returned. By this time, it was more difficult for Vern to get to the pool. And he didn't like it when I talked to other people, in fact became quite belligerent. I still managed to get him into the spa, and one day was able to talk to the husband we'd met the previous year. He told me his wife had started her slide into Alzheimers ten years previously, when she was only in her fifties. He also said this would be their last year at the park because everything was too hard for him.

The strain was beginning to tell on him but he always managed a smile when his wife was near.

Much of what I did during those three plus years and (certainly in the final year) was automatic. I never thought people were looking at me and wondering how I managed. People essentially were sympathetic, making comments of concern -- and often surprising me because I wasn't aware anyone noticed my caregiving problems.

At restaurants, people always offered to help me lift him from a seat. It depended on my mood whether I would accept or say, "Oh, I can do it. Thanks." I don't know whether it was my pride, stubbornness, or both when I wouldn't allow people to help me. As Vern became heavier and harder to move, I do admit that I allowed more people (usually men) to help.

I didn't realize what people saw.

We had gone to a special show at Knots Berry Farm one afternoon. Park attendants found a wheelchair for me to push Vern to the entrance at the show's end. Another attendant arrived in a golf cart to take us to our car. He was an older man about my age. When we arrived at our car he helped Vern into it. After he shut the door he came up to me and gave me a big hug. "Just hang in there," he said quietly. "You're doing great." What a neat demonstration of caring.

At our place near Palm Springs Vern loved to go to the pool on his scooter. This became a steadily more difficult task for me -- getting him into and out of the pool, sometimes to the pool shower, plus watching so he wouldn't run his scooter into the pool. Fortunately, friends at the pool helped me watch Vern when he was on his scooter.

One man said to me later, "You should have seen this poor woman trying to help her disabled husband at the pool." I told him that was me and he exclaimed, "You should have asked me for help."

Another time I had put Vern to bed one evening and slipped down to take a quick dip in the spa. A man sitting in the spa talked with me, then said, "You should see what is happening down the street. Some poor woman is trying to take care of her husband, and having quite a time getting him out of his chair and onto his walker." I laughed. "That woman is me."

After his death a woman said, "I watched you at the pool trying to give him a shower. I don't know how you did it."

As I look back I sometimes wonder also -- but know the good Lord gave me strength and the ability to persevere. Also, the knowledge that people did sympathize and did care meant a great deal.

An interesting situation I have encountered is the care of ex-husbands by ex-wives when the men develop incurable diseases.

The first such episode happened at least twenty years earlier between a female neighbor and her ex-husband. This had been a bitter divorce on the part of the wife because her husband had left her for another woman they both knew. When he got cancer, his new wife left him, and the ex-wife took him back and cared for him until his death. She said that he was the father of her children and she did for the children so they could visit their father and help care for him.

A second instance involved a couple who had been divorced for several years. They had five children during their marriage and did stay in contact because of the children. She remarried and then divorced, and moved to the mountains close to one of her sons. When her ex-husband became quite ill with terminal cancer she did not hesitate to take him into her home and care for him for almost two years. "I couldn't do anything else," she said. "He was the father of my children and we had always been friends. He needed me, and I stepped up to help."

The third case is the most interesting. After the couple divorced, the wife remarried. Her ex-husband and her new husband became friends. When the ex-husband got cancer and became ill, the new husband suggested he and his wife help the ex-husband. She agreed and the ex-husband lived with the ex-wife and her new husband throughout his illness.

Conclusion

Caregiving has existed for as long as the human race. However, because entire families lived together from young to old, there always was someone to care for the older person. Usually, this caregiver was the woman of the household. However, today a new caregiver has appeared -- a man who probably is caring for his ill spouse.

Caregivers have to be aware that when they find themselves in this new position it does change their lives. In many incidences, the change is gradual. The ill person can still do much for himself or herself. But as the disease progresses, more and more duties fall upon the caregiver from dressing and showering the ill person to dealing with moving the person from chair to walker or wheelchair.

Caregivers need to be aware that they will be tired and they need to think of themselves. They also need to retain as much contact with other people as possible. This contact is beneficial both for the loved one and for themselves.

And all caregivers need to know that other people not only are aware of their position but are willing to help in any way possible. Realization of this caring attitude on the part of others makes the caregiver role easier.

Some thoughts that kept me going:
"Duty alone is drudgery; duty with love is delight."

For young people caring for an older adult: "Kindness to the elderly brightens their sunset years."

For everyone going through this experience from caregiver to the one being cared for: "When wealth is gone, little is lost; when health is gone, something is lost; but when character is gone, all is lost."

Finally, two pieces of advice as you wonder why this is happening to you:

A person's religious beliefs often serve as a positive source of interpersonal strength. (advice from the American Association of Christian Counseling)

And if you wonder why this is happening to you: "Accept that both good and bad come to all of us. We do ourselves a disservice when we portray life as peaceful and happy all the time. Every season needs faith to get us through it."

CHAPTER TWO

FACTS ABOUT THE JOURNEY

The months became more difficult. Vern loved going out to eat -- but I began to get take-out instead. The stage shows and films he loved to attend, even church, became events of the past.

By October 2009, he was diagnosed with Stage 4 COPD. We were assigned a case worker who called regularly to find out how we were doing. This was also when I began to notice my increased workload. Making sure he didn't fall. Finding a walker for him to use if he had to go any distance. Helping him in and out of seats and the car. His eyes continued to fail to the point where he had a hard time reading his favorite page of the paper -- the comics.

I don't know when I started dressing him, or helping him in and out of the shower, or cutting up his food -- or finally showering him completely. It all becomes a blur -- but probably for over a year I was a caregiver in every sense of the word -- taking care of all Vern's needs. And he was hating my role in his life more and more -- because this was a proud man, so thrilled with the marriage we had, and now reduced to relying on me for everything.

That was brought totally to me when in the final days the man across from him in the skilled nursing facility said, "So you are Durlynn -- he calls for you all night long."

In October 2009, because of his difficult breathing, he finally was able to get oxygen (Stage 4 COPD) and a scooter to propel him around the house and outside.

Then January 2010 arrived, and with it the start of what the doctors called "Age Related Dementia." Why not just say Alzheimer's? But they never did say that until the end. Add in the fact he was losing his eyesight, and his resentment of all I had to do -- driving, yard work, pool maintenance, dressing and showering him. Yet, until the last six months he didn't want any outside help.

Life also changed for me. At first, it was in subtle ways. I watched Vern more closely because he had a habit of falling. He always had been a person who rushed to do something -- taking fast steps to get there as soon as possible. He could still get up and down stairs fairly well. Our home was built in a practical way so when we grew older we would need fewer stairs and obstacles. There were two steps from garage to house and three smaller steps from outside front yard to front door, but in the rear were many stairs to the backyard and pool area. Also, the pool did not have a rail at the steps because at the time of building we did not think it necessary.

How very necessary that pool rail became as the years slipped by. In those first two years after his fall, I was able to get him into the pool by use of a chair and myself carefully holding him. He loved the pool -- not to swim but to walk around. He had been the caretaker of the pool since we built the house and tried to maintain it the first year after he fell. Then that job along with scores of others fell to me.

Our mountain place was on a hillside which meant stairs were necessary to enter it, and downhill and uphill climbs were on much of the property. In February 2008, Vern fell down the hillside twice -- both times because he was rushing! I realized I had to keep an eye on him whenever we were outside.

Stairs were built to enter our RV which was parked at a resort near the coast. Whenever Vern went up or down the stairs at our Palm Springs area home, guess where I was? Right behind or ahead of him.

When the caregiving journey begins you'll have many things to consider. First, you will have to realize the extent of your caregiving. This will depend on the condition of the one for whom you are caring. Several people interviewed talked about the early care of the loved one, who still could do many things for himself or herself. This person could be left at home with no fears of an accident happening. This person could still dress and shower himself or herself.

But as the loved one became increasingly frail, the caregiving duties also increased. This is when decisions have to be made about the best place for care (which will be covered in Chapter Three). One interviewee said, "I was always Daddy's girl, and promised him I would always take care of him. But when he became so ill I knew I couldn't do it and keep the job I had. Fortunately, I had a sister and brother-in-law who took over -- willingly!"

You'll see two terms used for caregivers: informal caregiver and family caregiver. This simply means usually a family member or close family friend is the caregiver. These are unpaid people providing care. As the American population ages, the number of caregivers and the demands placed on them will grow. These caregivers help with a multitude of things, including: grocery shopping, house cleaning, cooking, shopping for other items, paying bills, giving medicine, toileting, bathing, dressing, and eating.

Paid caregivers also are available, either through private funds or government in-home support groups. When looking for a paid caregiver, examine their backgrounds and be sure they are bonded. Horror stories abound when not checking on these people and later discovering they are stealing from the older person. However, if you are the chief caregiver and these people come into your home under your supervision, you may not have a problem. In-home caregivers can free you to leave or work. They can support you anywhere from one or two days a week to a full time five days. If you simply need someone to shower your loved one and perhaps stay an hour or two while you do errands, you can have that support half a day, two or three days a week. You work out the schedule that best fits your needs.

Finally, many localities throughout the United States have Adult Day Care Centers (although with restricted budgets these government funded programs may not now be available). The client usually is provided with transportation, a day at the center, and a hot lunch. You also can drop them off on your way to an appointment or work. Activities include exercise programs, sing-a-longs, therapy, and most of all social contact. When your loved one is around others and can talk and laugh, it makes their life more complete.

Caregiving can become a full time job twenty-four hours a day seven days a week, with no rest times in between the journey. Or it becomes a watching and helping journey as the loved one either stays at his or her own home or enters a rehabilitation/nursing facility.

Three Ways of Caring

Mine has been a journey in all three ways to care for a loved one. My mother died at fifty-seven years-old after years of illness, either brought on as real illness or by her hypochondriac ways. As an only grandchild, I took over my grandmother's care when my uncle and father died. My last journey was Vern's care. Each of the three was handled in a different way.

My mother always lived in her own place -- going from a house when she and my stepfather divorced to apartments -- many apartments during six years. I am an only child, my parents having divorced when I was fourteen. In the forties and fifties, I automatically lived with my mother, thus moving with her and my stepfather to the San Francisco Bay area when he was transferred. Fortunately, during my mother's later illnesses she lived in her own apartment.

When my mother divorced her second husband, they agreed to sell their house. She found what she called a "darling apartment" and my husband and I moved her into it. This was the beginning of a series of apartments for her. She still could drive, so was able to do her own shopping, appointments, and social activities.

Major surgery started her downhill spiral. At that time, she needed 24/7 care after the surgery but could only retain a day nurse. At night, I'd get my three children ready for bed, kiss my husband goodbye and do the night duty. I arose at five to go home and get my husband's breakfast, fix his lunch, and get him off to work. Then came breakfast for the children and lunches for the older two. The youngest went back to nana's with me until the day nurse arrived.

Then she moved again. By this time, I was taking her to doctor's appointments and helping with shopping. I was in contact with her either by telephone or personally every day. I complicated this routine by returning to college to finish my degree. (When I quit college at nineteen my parents despaired I would never return. I knew better!).

Things progressed to the point where she rarely left her apartment. I helped as much as I could and called or went to see her every day. Except one day. It was the day after Thanksgiving and a cousin of my husband's arrived at my doorstep(unannounced) with family. I hadn't called my mother because of lunch and visiting with them. At 4:30 p.m. a neighbor who visited her each afternoon called, "Come quick. Something's wrong with your mother."

I went and found her dead on her couch at fifty-seven years old.

Thus, my care for my mother was in her own home the entire time.

This was not the case for my grandmother. Her oldest son (my uncle) died of a heart attack at fifty-one-years old. My dad was five years younger than his brother and died at forty-nine years old. I am an only grandchild on my dad's side of the family. Therefore, long before he died, we talked about the possibility of me taking care of my grandmother if anything happened to him.

I agreed that my dad's will would leave everything to my grandmother (in order to take care of her) and the proverbial dollar to me. That was fine with me because I knew how worried he was about her care. Then he remarried (a third wife). When he died, his wife challenged the will and won, gaining the money. My dad's attorney had not only written my dad's will but also was the wife's attorney who overturned that original will!

She promised to take care of my grandmother, and because they were in San Diego five hundred miles from me, I thought it was a good idea.

At first, my grandmother was happy with my stepmother's care. Aside from eye problems (macular degeneration), my grandmother was very healthy, having walked everywhere during her lifetime. My stepmother decided grandmother should fly to visit me (she was ninety-four years old). She thoroughly enjoyed her first airplane trip. Little did I know what my stepmother had in mind. While grandmother was visiting me, my stepmother moved her to a retirement home.

This wasn't all bad because my grandmother's eyes were rapidly failing and we were worried about her living alone. But the retirement home was miles from her church, her major social activity.

Grandmother became upset with my stepmother and decided I had to take over her financial obligations right away. Fortunately, it was summer, so my family and I went to San Diego to transfer everything. Grandmother was happy about her new arrangements and then...

She contacted shingles and never recovered her health. She now was ninety-six and seemed to let go when she realized I would take care of her the rest of her life.

The first thing I had to do was find a convalescent hospital for her. As will be explained in Chapter Three, that isn't easy. However, I found one that was clean, cheerful and appeared to be a good choice . . . until she broke a hip. Then I found another convalescent hospital. By then, I realized the five hundred mile separation wasn't easy for either of us. The key to nursing homes is regular visits, and of course I couldn't do that.

With her doctor's blessing, I found a convalescent hospital near my house in the San Francisco Bay Area and went down to fly her to our town. Because she was coming to my hometown, she couldn't understand why she couldn't live with my family. However, our three bedroom, one bath house with three children wasn't big enough (my daughter certainly didn't want to be with her brothers in one bedroom).

A convalescent hospital within half a mile was perfect. I'd visit either on the way home from work or after work and two of my children also visited (one did not like hospital visits and I wouldn't make him go). I was in touch with the home the entire time my grandmother lived there, and because they never knew when I would arrive I had no worries about her care. I did visit almost every day for three plus years.

My grandmother's was the second method of caregiving -- certainly easier than at home but also time consuming if I wanted to do it correctly.

Most of this book will cover the third method -- the in-home care of the loved one -- which is 24/7 duty no matter what anyone says. The two other caregiving roles also will be continued in other chapters.

Looking at Statistics

Statistics demonstrate the extent of caregiving in the U. S. The National Alliance for Caregiving and American Association of Retired People (AARP) found that 44.4 million Americans age eighteen or older are providing unpaid care to an adult. Interestingly, the typical caregiver is a forty-six-year-old woman with some college education who works and also spends more than twenty hours per week caring for her mother who lives nearby. You notice this falls into the role I had with my mother. Almost seven in ten (69%) caregivers say they care for one person with the average length of caregiving at 4.3 years. (It was over six years for my mother and grandmother, 3.3 years for my husband.) Most caregivers are married or living with a partner (62%) and most have worked and managed caregiving responsibilities at the same time (74%).

These statistics add up to a multitude of problems faced by caregivers -- and, if a family with children is a part of it, some crucial problems for the family as well.

Stages of Caregiving (as given in Several References)

Stage 1. I may help a relative soon.
Stage 2. I am beginning to help.
Stage 3. I am helping.
Stage 4. I am still helping.
Stage 5. My role is changing (becoming more time consuming.)
Stage 6. My caregiving has ended.

Along the way, most caregivers find themselves with several challenges. Almost sixty percent either work or have worked while providing the care. They have found they had to make adjustments to their work schedules, or in some cases even had to give up work entirely.

Male caregivers are more likely to work full or part time jobs compared to fifty-five to sixty-six percent of females.

One of the most interesting (and obviously loving) caregivers I met was a professional woman who brought both her mother and her developmentally disabled adult sister from the East Coast to the West Coast because she was concerned about their care.

Her mother had become quite frail and this woman felt her sister's care was too much for her mother. She brought them both to her home. "I'd never think of having them anywhere else," she said.

Then her sister became ill and went to the hospital. This professional woman, who had a demanding job, managed to balance her periodic visits to her sister's hospital with care of her mother and still do an outstanding performance on her job.

Personally, I think because her job involved care of people, she had more than enough empathy to accomplish three tasks and remain strongly committed to all of them.

Most caregivers help relatives, with eighty percent of care recipients over fifty years old. One quarter of caregivers helping someone fifty or older report this person is suffering from Alzheimer's, dementia, or other mental confusion.

From these statistics and examples, you can see that caregivers have unmet needs and often are just plain exhausted.

Needs along the Journey

One of the major things you need to know on this journey is that you are not alone. Many times I realized my caregiving wasn't as hard as that of other people. In restaurants, I watched women or men with loved ones far less mobile than my husband. They were managing and usually smiling. I heard about women with husbands who had strokes. These men went home to be in hospital beds and needed constant care. Not only did these women have a difficult caregiving job, but their husbands often did not want outside help.

When I saw or heard these stories, I'd tell myself I really didn't have it that bad -- and would believe it! Because it was true.

> *The greatest proof of the ease of my "normal" caregiving compared to others was when I met Mrs. J. She was a lovely woman in her early fifties who didn't display the emotional trauma of her life. Her son was diagnosed with muscular dystrophy when he was five.*
>
> *"He was active and mobile until he was fourteen," she said. "Then he went into a wheelchair but still managed to get a B. A. in history summa cum lauda." She paused, then added, "The whole thing about this was that he wasn't supposed to live that long. My husband and I went on that theory, expecting him to die any minute. My son is still going strong at thirty-two."*
>
> *Ten years previously Mrs. J had her double whammy. Her husband was diagnosed with cancer. He had several surgeries and lived for two years at home.*
>
> *Consequently, Mrs. J had a double caregiving experience -- caring both for her son and for her husband during that two year period. She was quick to add that her older son, who had not married, moved back home to help when he could. However, most of the caregiving fell on Mrs. J.*

Most of us are not aware there are many people like Mrs. J -- caregivers with both spouse and child or spouse and parent ailing and needing care. Theirs is the more than twenty-four hour job -- and one that might not stop for many years.

Due to the amount of caregivers in our society today, resources have been developed from several different organizations and groups to help you deal with this new phenomenon in your lives. You and I might think we can cope with any situation, but this cannot always be the case. Caregiving is a special existence, and a great deal more than anyone can envision.

An excellent resource was developed by The National Family Caregivers Association and National Alliance for Caregiving. Their concise list gives you an idea of what to expect both for your caregiving responsibilities and for yourself. Their contact information is in the Resources section of this book.

CAREGIVING

➤ itself is a multi-dimensional puzzle, meaning all kinds of things to provide for a person in need. It may mean providing 24-hour care for someone who can't dress, feed, go to the bathroom, or think for himself or herself. Or it may be an emotional roller coaster because a diagnosed condition has not exhibited debilitating symptoms -- yet!

➤ can go on for a few years or for a lifetime. It means for the caregiver re-evaluation of finances and job opportunities as well as making compromises.

➤ is learning how to work with doctors and other healthcare professionals so they treat you as an important member of your loved one's healthcare team.

➤ is worrying about what's wrong with dad, mom or spouse, and wanting the truth.

➤ includes learning about wheelchairs, lifts, little gadgets to help with tasks.

➤ is wondering why no one ever asks how you are.

➤ is dreaming about being alone in your own house.

➤ involves learning about Medicare, Medicaid, social security, and other public programs.

➤ is learning what it means to die with dignity and make sure that your loved one's wishes will be honored.

➤ is the joy you feel when your spouse says he/she feels good today

➤ is the relief you feel when your mother decides it's time to move out of the big house and into an assisted living complex.

➤ is hard work and pain.

➤ is loving, giving, sharing, accepting and learning new things and going on, and on.

➤ has lots of questions and few answers and it is being out of the mainstream.

➤ is all these things and a whole lot more.

Keep this list handy during all of your caregiving. Refer to it often, especially during periods of frustration, anger, or weariness. Some of you already can recognize everything on this list (I could when reading it). For others, your time has only just begun.

You may anticipate what will happen and think you are ready to face this new situation. No one understands the deep involvement of caregiving. When I took care of my mother and grandmother I was in my late twenties/early thirties. None of my husband's and my friends were involved with these types of situations. Consequently, I never thought to mention to anyone about my new circumstances. It was just another part of my life.

But caregiving did become a major part of my life. This is where duty is a component. Not to care for my mother or grandmother was not an option. It was just another task as I continued to take care of my husband and children. And it didn't stop me from being involved in other activities. I managed to be president of the PTA, then go back to finish my B. A. After my mother died, I still had to care for grandmother, which was when I brought her north to be near us. At that time, I started a new teaching job. I had earned my teaching credential through hard work and was offered a job I couldn't turn down.

Oh yes, about that time my husband took a severe fall at work and was disabled the remainder of his life. Fortunately, he was only in his forties and could care for himself -- and did until his death at fifty-eight.

> *The biggest problem for caregivers is their unmet needs, as enumerated by the National Family Caregivers Association and the National Alliance for Caregivers. These needs include:*
> ✓ *Finding time for yourself (35%), managing emotional and physical stress (29%), and balancing work and family responsibilities (29%).*
> ✓ *Thirty percent say they need help keeping the person they care for safe and finding easy activities to do with the person they care for.*
> ✓ *Twenty-two percent say they need help talking with doctors and other healthcare professionals or making end-of-life decisions.*

Don't be afraid to ask for help. My husband had a case worker and a social worker (we are members of Kaiser Permanente). When I became absolutely frazzled or didn't know what I should do next, I called them. I didn't call often, which meant when I did call they immediately responded -- and I felt better after that call.

Above everything else, you need to know you are not alone. Millions of people are caregivers. Excellent internet sites (see end) show you how to cope. Numerous books can answer your questions. Take advantage of all known sources -- and continue to treat yourself carefully.

Conclusion

You're now faced with some big questions about what you will do next for your loved one. If your parent or parents are still living in their own home or apartment, you have to decide how best you can help them stay where they are (at least for a while). You may have to help with shopping, cleaning, or driving to their appointments. And you have to be aware there might come a time when they have to move to a more secure environment.

Don't feel guilty if you cannot care for your loved one in your home. There are excellent skilled nursing facilities, assisted living facilities, and rehabilitation facilities. That is covered in the next chapter.

And if you are caring for your spouse, a parent, or another older adult in your home, accept and learn all you can about in-home caregiving. The caregiving will not be easy. You must be aware of your own unmet needs even as you expend a huge amount of energy in your caregiving role.

This final note from the National Family Caregivers Association and the National Alliance for Caregiving: Next time you feel guilty for even thinking about taking a break, remember it is only partially for your benefit. Your loved one will reap a great deal of the benefit as well.

CHAPTER THREE

THE JOURNEY'S MANY BYROADS

As Vern's health declined, several people suggested that perhaps he should go to a long term care facility. But I knew that would be an impossibility for him. He loved being at home. I'd take him out on the deck, and even with his poor eyesight and hearing, he still enjoyed the nature around him. In the winter, I'd sit him on the south side of the house where he could bask in the warm sunshine. This was his home -- with his own bed, recliner chair and dinette table. He was accustomed to them. Proof of what a long term care facility would have done to his emotional and mental state were the nineteen days he spent in the hospital and skilled nursing at the end.

At that final time I had no choice. After emergency services in Palm Springs (where we were when he fell), he was placed in the hospital -- first in the cardiac unit because of an irregular heartbeat and then in acute care because of the swift arrival of Alzheimer's and his increasingly acute COPD. During his nine days at the Palm Springs facility I was with him from eight to ten hours a day with the exception of two days when his daughter from Phoenix took over. My presence helped him through those days.

Then he was moved to a facility in Stockton. I was staying with my son and his wife during that time but now had other needs -- mail to pick up, bills to pay, and some important doctor appointments for myself. I didn't see Vern as much but my two sons and their wives went in every day -- and weekends were full of family from Fresno plus grandchildren. However, I could tell he missed my constant visits and disliked lying in bed. His decline did not take long. Nineteen days after he went to emergency he had passed away.

Caregiving decisions are very difficult at every stage of an illness.

From the beginning of your caregiving, it is vital you get as much information as possible about all stages of an illness as well as its progression. I was in my late twenties/early thirties when my mother and grandmother went through their illnesses so I knew very little about caregiving or illness. But I learned quickly. That time period was over forty years ago, so life and resultant care were much different.

In those days, the only facilities for older people were convalescent homes and hospitals. There were no retirement homes or communities. Convalescent was really another word for "Put them somewhere and we'll pay a little attention to their needs."

Consequently, when I looked for facilities for my grandmother I was appalled at where older people were lodged. I entered place after place that reeked of urine and had residents either strapped into wheelchairs or lying in their beds. I couldn't believe the treatment and vowed I would look until I found a decent place for my grandmother (remember I lived five hundred miles from her).

When it came to where my husband would be almost forty years later there was no question -- he would stay in our home. My greatest problem as he grew more feeble was that he didn't want anyone else dressing and showering him.

But you do need to be aware of how to handle the next step toward whatever type of caregiving you decide upon.

Stella Mora Henry in her book **The Eldercare Handbook** *talks about signs to watch for that will help with your decisions. These start when your loved one (probably parents, a parent or a grandparent) are still living in their own home or apartment.*

✓ *Personal Care. How is their personal hygiene -- bathing, messy hair, soiled clothing, etc?*
✓ *Housekeeping -- How does the house look -- dirty dishes, piled up laundry, etc?*
✓ *Meals and Appetite -- Can they fix meals? Do they have a decreased appetite etc?*
✓ *Memory -- Do they forget important things like appointments, how to use telephone or TV, etc?*
✓ *Communication -- Do they have difficulty finding words, writing legibly, etc?*
✓ *Mobility -- Do they walk with a slower pace, have difficulty climbing stairs, fall frequently, etc?*
✓ *Depression -- Are they increasingly anxious or irritable, less interested in family and friends?*
✓ *Medication -- Do they take their medications correctly or either overuse or forget?*
✓ *Finances -- You must do this. Quickly look around the house to be sure there aren't any unpaid bills, unopened mail, unexplained credit card charges, etc.*
✓ *Driving -- Here's a hard one. There will come a time when you have to insist they can no longer drive. Go with them to monitor how they drive -- turning, speeding, difficulty parking, etc.--then you may have to break the bad news.*

If you start to think about alternative living arrangements when you first observe these signs, you will be ahead when you have to take over the myriad duties to keep your loved one safe. Those same signs can be used for those of you uncertain about what is happening to your spouse.

My husband felt confident about our banking so I didn't question him about paying bills or check book balances. However, shortly after we returned from our Branson trip he wrote me a check for another account. When I went to deposit it the teller told me it was almost illegible. I talked about my husband and how I hated to take that responsibility away from him. She said I'd better do it because it was a miracle none of the checks he had written had not been returned.

I quietly talked to him about what was said and was surprised when he agreed to let me take over financial responsibilities. I later gathered he had been concerned -- couldn't see well with his deteriorating eyesight and just didn't want to admit something he knew was inevitable.

He was wonderful about this. Can't say what other people might do in similar circumstances.

Coming to grips with signs of increasing frailty early will help you later. My mother never had problems with her checkbook. And remember, I took over for my grandmother as soon as she put me on her account. I think she was glad she didn't have to do it, just like my husband.

All this is necessary as we move toward caregiving.

Denial Enters the Journey

In many ways, I'm glad I'm an only child when it came to the decisions for my mother and grandmother. One of the biggest problems you'll encounter is denial. You are around your parent (s) and know what is happening. If your sibling lives miles away and visits seldom, he or she might not agree if you decide to move your parent (s) into a more secure environment. This is called denial.

Denial is a defense mechanism. It may be your way of first coping, and it certainly is often the coping mechanism for siblings (etc) who are a long distance. Confronting this denial does two things: (1) gives you and the family time to absorb what is going to happen with the changes of your loved one, and (2) gives a chance to regroup for the task ahead.

Perhaps you are watching your parent do some strange things -- not dressing properly or forgetting to pay bills or any number of other little things. You tell yourself it really isn't important -- but sooner or later you have to admit changes are occurring. With Vern, the dementia didn't set in for at least two years. My concern was his falling -- which continued to worsen.

What is fascinating about dementia is that a loved one can act perfectly normal when someone is visiting -- as long as the visit is short. Maybe a sibling is visiting and can't understand what you are talking about regarding deteriorating mental capacity. Remember, he or she doesn't see the entire 24/7 picture.

I doubt that I really tried to cover up anything that was happening to Vern. However, the few people who visited, as well as his daughters, asked few questions nor seemed to see the reality. In retrospect, they now tell me they noticed all kinds of things, but never bothered to mention anything to me.

If you are in a long distance situation and notice changes in your loved one when you visit, be sure to tell the caregiver. That way the caregiver won't think he or she is simply imagining all this.

Journey to a New Place

The reality of our modern lives is that not all people can do caregiving in their homes. No one should feel guilty about this. My mother, although becoming increasingly frail, still was able to be in her own home, although I wondered when I would have to move her to a more secure place. My grandmother entered a facility while still five hundred miles from me. I had no choice. She couldn't stay in her retirement apartment. The management would not allow it.

When you make a choice to move a loved one to a more secure environment, you must do a thorough visit to find the right place.

X's mother was steadily going downhill, with a diagnosis of Alzheimers looming. Her mother would wander away from the retirement home in which she lived, to the point where the manager told X her mother had to go somewhere else.

"This was in the day when there weren't very many nice convalescent homes," X said. "And the best one in town had a waiting list."

X put her mother on the waiting list. Then she tried to find a more than adequate facility while awaiting the next move. That was difficult because her mother continued to wander away from a facility with some terrible consequences. She rode a bus to the other side of town and became totally lost (police picked her up). She even ended up in a strange apartment.

It took X several months to finally get her mother in the best care facility in the area.

"I had two small boys and I was working full time," X said. "A convalescent home was the only answer. But it had to be quality care and environment. That took almost a year."

When you decide to find a care home you must allow yourself at least one solid week, although two search weeks are better. This is not always possible. When I had to find a place for my grandmother, my time was limited. I saw several horrors before I was lucky to find a clean place with no odors and an obvious concern for patients.

But my elation turned to frustration in three months. A staff member left the rails on one side of her bed down. Grandmother proceeded to get up, fall down and break her hip. Please remember, I still was new at this procedure and didn't realize it was the facility's fault and they should have paid for everything that happened to her after the fall.

Instead of realizing the facility's fault and attempting a law suit, I just wanted her away from the situation. When she left the hospital, where she had been taken after the fall, I had a beautiful new home for her -- the most expensive in the San Diego area. This was good for my peace of mind (in those days expensive was $800.00 a month!).

When I was ready to move her north, I again visited every facility in my area. I could take the time because I wasn't going to move her until I found the right place. They had just built a two hundred fifty bed convalescent facility half a mile from my house. It appeared perfect for her and proved to meet all my expectations. I felt very good about bringing her close to our family at last.

As soon as your loved one becomes ill, frail, or on a downward cycle, become familiar with what Medicare and Medicaid has to offer. I'm certainly glad I knew.

Essentially, my grandmother had enough money for me to pay her monthly bills for about two years. Remember, my stepmother had taken the money that was supposed to come to my grandmother in my dad's will. I asked the manager at the facility what I was going to do when her money ran out. He replied, " Don't worry. Your grandmother can go on Medicaid and will receive the same care."

Shortly after that conversation she had to go to Medicaid -- and found his words were true. Her care remained the same until her death.

You can find a good home for your loved one -- and never feel guilty if that is all you can do. As long as you visit as often as possible, you can feel you are caring and doing everything possible. (I usually did it daily, even if it was for a short time. I also went at different times.)

An interview with Victor Reyes, Admissions Coordinator, Wagner Heights Nursing and Rehabilitation Center in Stockton, California (where Vern was at the end so I can vouch for the excellent care) talked to me about his procedures when a family is searching for a facility for their loved one.

He said he and the staff try to treat the family and the patient with complete respect and love. Before admittance, he sits down with the family and patient (if possible) to talk about the facility and what to expect. They walk around the facility to view the rooms and activities.

He and the staff recognize that this is a transition and hard on both family and patient. They try to make that transition as easy as possible.

"We need to put ourselves in their place," he said. "That makes all the difference." Then he added that the important key to success is love. "Love is all of it," he concluded.

The Journey at Home

If you make the decision to care for your loved one at home, and this is certainly the case for spouses, then you have to take several factors into consideration.

Learn all you can about your loved one's illness. Ask the doctor and health care professionals about everything related to the illness and your responsibilities. NEVER be afraid to ask questions.

Don't be afraid to make demands. My husband was having a terrible time breathing, yet couldn't get oxygen due to Medicare rules. When he entered Stage 4 COPD I began to ask for (demand) his oxygen. The doctor and case worker saw my point and advocated until Vern received oxygen.

Learn all you can about Medicare and Medicaid or whatever your health plan may be. Find out what it covers and what it does not cover.

Find out about end-of-life options. If your loved one has cancer, heart disease, Parkinson's, or any other terminal illness, hospice may be there for you and your loved one. But Vern had COPD and hospice was not an option for him. Palliative care was available but my husband did not want someone else to dress and shower him so refused that option.

Adult Day Care was discussed in Chapter Two. If you need time to do errands, go to appointments or just relax, OR if you have a part or full time job, this is an excellent resource IF the person for whom you are caring is mobile. It gives them a social experience instead of being at home all the time. Three other options so you aren't as burdened are in-home support, palliative care, and later Hospice.

In-home support agencies are available in most communities, although that service usually provided by state financing, is disappearing as state budgets become tighter. If your parent (s), spouse, or other loved one is on Medicaid you will receive these services at no charge. You also can investigate to see how much you need to pay if not on Medicaid because charge is usually based on income.

The in-home support person, usually a nurse's aide, comes in two to three days a week and can help with bathing, bed changing, feeding, or any other type of care necessary to make the loved one more comfortable.

My suggestions to Vern about in-home support care were rejected. He didn't want anyone else to dress and shower him (two of my biggest tasks). I suggested some lesser tasks like feeding him lunch or watching him while I went out with my granddaughters. Fortunately, the woman who did my housecleaning had a nursing background. He liked her and finally agreed to have her occasionally with him. She told me later he seemed to enjoy their lunchtime conversations because he could talk about the Bible and Jesus.

Palliative care focuses on helping patients with their pain and symptoms to make the most of their lives as they deal with a serious illness. It is about living right now with illnesses like cancer, heart disease, diabetes or COPD. Included in the services are counseling, rehabilitation, and managing the pain and suffering. This care was offered to Vern at a late stage of his COPD but he already was beyond any type of rehabilitation or counseling -- very settled into his present circumstances.

Most people and their at-home caregiver would appreciate knowing more about Palliative Care and what it covers. Take advantage of the services offered because it will help you as well as your loved one. Among their services is the managing of the complicated health system. Another service is improving the quality of life for the patient through therapy and activities. A comment made by a case manager was, "Those needing palliative care don't realize they have a right to care focused on improving function and quality of life."

That quality of life issue is the main part of the service. Although palliative care is quite new, studies show it is making a difference. Patients who have elected it have lived three plus months more and have understood their medical regimes more than regular patients. It is still in its infancy and needs more study. However, if your loved one is seriously ill, talk to your physician about having a consultation. It can improve serious conditions. And think what it does for the caregiver.

Hospice is for care as the end of life approaches. This care option not only gives care for the patient but also some respite for the caregiver. The mission of Hospice is to provide comprehensive medical and compassionate care, counseling and support to terminally ill patients and their families. Hospice is not concerned about ability to pay because they are there to educate families about making the end of life the best possible experience for the loved one and the family involved. They collaborate with health care providers and the public to promote quality end-of-life care. Vern had Hospice for the last two days of his life when we made the decision to only make him comfortable at the end.

In my case, I needed to learn more about Hospice. When Vern finally went on the program, I assumed they were paying for everything (he was in skilled nursing). Not so. He immediately went on private care. Hospice had been recommended by the doctor earlier but they had not contacted me until a Friday. He became worse on Saturday, which was when they allowed Hospice to come in.

If I had known what I know now, I would have asked that he be released to our home and then have Hospice. Then he would have been at home at the end -- but I did not know.

As a caregiver take these tips to heart:

> Take charge of your life, even with your loved one's illness or disability.
> When people offer to help, accept the offer and support what they can do.
> Educate yourself about your loved one's condition. Information is empowering, especially when talking to healthcare professionals.
> Be open to technologies and ideas that can help your loved one keep his or her   independence.
> Trust your instincts. Most of the time they will lead you in the right direction.
> Seek support of other caregivers. Know you are not alone.
> Learn to delegate some of your responsibilities. You do not have to do everything by yourself -- communicate your needs to family, neighbors, friends. You'll be amazed how much people really want to help, but often are afraid to ask.
> You are in for a long journey -- but with the right attitude and information you can succeed.

Conclusion

Be aware of the stages toward caregiving for your loved one. Be aware of the signs toward possible disability or frailness. If you are prepared, it will make the journey easier.

Denial is part of the process for you and family members. Recognize what is happening to your loved one. Also, understand how siblings living a distance from you may not realize all that is happening.

You have to make the decision about your loved one's next move. Will it be a stay in his or her own home, a move to a long term care facility, or a move to your home? These decisions must be carefully considered -- not only for the loved one but for you and how much you (and if you have a family, the family members) can do.

When considering a long term care facility visit as many as possible at different times of the day. And if you decide to place your loved one in a facility, be sure to visit as often as possible and at different times of the day.

If you decide to keep your loved one in your home, learn all you can about Medicare, Medicaid, health care for the elderly and options you may have for respite care.

Knowledge will help you and your loved one survive this new challenge in both of your lives.

CHAPTER FOUR

A PARENT/CHILD, CHILD/PARENT JOURNEY

When I received the phone call from my grandmother to come to San Diego right away because she wanted me to take over her finances, I wasn't surprised. My step-mother had said she would care for my grandmother, but I know she never expected my grandmother to live a long time. Now my grandmother was concerned that my step-mother wouldn't take care of her and turned to me, her only grandchild. I went to the bank with her as well as the stock brokers office and officially became a co-signer on all her accounts, with my step-mother removed.

This seemed an awesome responsibility for a younger person (late twenties/early thirties), but I thought grandmother would remain in her retirement home apartment for many years. That was not the case. It seemed like overnight things happened to her -- first shingles which in the late sixties had no shots to alleviate the pain. Shingles were her turning point and before I left San Diego I had to place her in a convalescent hospital. Her eyes had deteriorated to the point where she could hardly see. The retirement home management told me she could no longer remain there.

I had little time to find a decent convalescent hospital, and just hoped the place I found would be all right. She didn't even resist going. It seemed at ninety-seven years-old that she was ready to rely on me completely. It was a good thing I was only in my late twenties, never realizing how much I would have to do.

Caregiving gives an entirely different dimension to the parent/child relationship -- one few of us expect to experience.

I've been in the caregiver role many times and always wondered why the Lord gave it to me when I've never been particularly sympathetic to illness (my children complained about my reactions when they were sick). My divorced mother was ill for years. Although she did not live with me, I was an only child, so she depended on me, as enumerated in earlier chapters.

Then came the care for my grandmother on my father's side, as described previously. Her two sons died early -- my uncle at fifty-one and my dad at forty-nine; my grandmother lived to be one-hundred-two. Her last five years were spent in the convalescent hospital. In her final year, she already was in a different world, most times not even knowing me.

Both my mother-in-laws were ill at the end of their lives -- and both husbands did the majority of caregiving for them.

Finally, there was my second husband who gave so much to my life. What could I do but care totally for him when he began to fail?

Each of the above persons was extremely independent. My grandmother had raised two sons by herself, and kept her own house until well into her nineties. Ironically, in her late nineties when I agreed to take over her finances and care, she totally became dependent on me. I had two independent mothers-in-law. Yet, their lives suddenly changed.

One day my first husband and I went to his mother's house to take her to dinner. We knew something was wrong when she said she'd rather we brought in "take-out." We knew our role had changed for her.

When Vern's mother broke her arm and was recuperating at our house, she said, "It's really nice here. I'd better get home or I just might stay forever." I knew our next role would come soon.

And my mother? I don't know when I took over the parent role but feel it probably was after she divorced her second husband.

As I look back, I am happy that much of the care for my mother and grandmother happened when I was in my late twenties and early thirties. At that point, I had three children, had decided to return to college to finish my B. A., was working a small do-at-home job, and of course running my household. Our house was in a typical fifties/sixties tract (called housing development now) with three bedrooms and one bath -- not a place to bring another adult. None of our friends were in any caregiving situations -- all having lively parents.

My mother loved doctors and loved surgeries -- a true hypochondriac. This was the major reason I became the parent and her the child who needed me at varying times during her five year downhill spiral. She went from driving to having me take her to doctor appointments or go shopping with her. Then she simply called me to get her groceries -- or she would call the store to bring the groceries to her.

And she kept finding new doctors because she was certain her old ones were not listening to her. I could understand that. After one surgery, when I was having trouble finding nursing help for her, the doctor said, "Well, she's your mother and your problem. You figure out what to do."

In that instance, I went to her apartment each night after I put the children to bed. Then I was up at five a. m. to drive home and get my husband off to work and the children off to school -- all with good breakfasts.

I either went to her apartment or called her each day -- never missed if I could help it. It wasn't that she was demanding -- just seemed to need me all the time for big or little problems.

As I said previously, it was lucky I was in my late twenties/early thirties and could do all this and more. What is the comment? Thank goodness for youth!

From Present to Future

I'm sure parents aren't any happier relying on their children than the children are to have these new responsibilities. And this reversal is the major problem.

Right now, you can't imagine your parents or even grandparents relying totally on you. Most of them are still driving and probably maintaining their own homes or apartments. Perhaps you have parents who spend the summer at home and the winter in a community in the south or west. You think nothing will ever change.

Think about your own parents or grandparents. They most likely are as independent as the examples mentioned above. Probably they own their own homes -- maintaining these homes as you grew and expecting to keep these homes the rest of their lives. They've put energy into their property and can't imagine their lives in another place. Other parents and grandparents have made the transition to smaller places, many times in a retirement community. They still live independently and plan to do this for the remainder of their lives.

Worry exemplifies the start of caregiving and stays for the entire time. CC was an only child with separated parents (they had never divorced because of her mother's Roman Catholic beliefs). CC described her mother as "very spunky" and always wanting to do things by herself. Mother, now in her eighties, lived in her own house and didn't want to move into a retirement facility, no matter how much CC begged.

When Mother turned ninety, CC was more worried about her. Mother was beginning to show the signs of aging; not caring for herself, or the house like the past. As Mother's frailty increased, CC decided she had to move her to assisted living. Mother fought this all the way, but CC could see no alternative. She was certain her mother would fall at some point and break a bone, or simply forget the stove had been lit.

Against her mother's wishes but because she was so worried, CC moved her mother to a "beautiful" assisted living home. Mother was so upset she gave up, refusing to participate in activities or come out of her room. Nine months later mother died.

CC misses her mother a great deal but feels her mother's death was a great relief to her and her husband. "And now she can be spunky again!" CC says with a sad smile.

Driving -- here's a major hurdle for your parent (s) and for you. As an older adult, I know my reactions are slower than in the past, and am well aware that sometime in the future I may have to give up driving -- just hope it won't be for ten years or more! For this reason, I moved from my lovely house in the mountains to the town where my sons live -- a place that has decent public transportation.

But too many older people refuse to admit their driving habits may be dangerous. Their children must be the ones to suggest less driving, or even giving up the license.

> *Vern was typical of the older person who didn't want to give up his license. His eyes were deteriorating which meant I didn't want him on the freeway, nor our winding mountain roads. I knew he was getting less certain of himself through two incidents.*
>
> *We often travel I-5 to Southern California which entails a trip over the Grapevine. He had little problem going up the grade. However, one day after we had stopped at the rest area before descending, he said, "Could you keep on driving?" I knew he no longer felt confident driving the downhill portion.*
>
> *The second incident occurred quite frequently toward the end of his driving. He would try to drive the freeway, then suddenly pull to the side of the road. "You take over," he'd say. No other explanation, but I knew why.*
>
> *Actually, having him cede his license was harder. He no longer drove after his severe fall in November 2007, but he couldn't give up that license. I kept telling him our insurance rates would go down but he didn't listen. Finally, he gave up the license for an ID card about nine months before he died.*

The license is a symbol of independence that parents hate to give up. Can you blame them? That license is their demonstration they can take care of themselves. When it goes they know they have to rely on someone else. (By the way, driving is a privilege not a right.)

As you and your parents or grandparents move forward, the present becomes a future none of you envisioned. You are going to have to face that reality.

Facing Reality

An interesting phenomenon often happens when the older person decides to rely totally on another person (spouse, child, perhaps grandchild). He or she now relies completely. It's almost like they have given up on the life they once knew. This is the time when caregivers need to know their responsibility is not only to do the necessities, but also to make the person for whom they are caring feel life is still worthwhile.

When I brought my grandmother north she relied completely on me and the staff of the nursing home. Her reliance on me started when she got shingles while I was at her retirement apartment. She wanted me to bathe her, dress her, help with her feeding. I knew then that I was going to have to put her in what then was called a nursing home. She no longer was able to take care of herself -- plus I felt she really didn't care to do it any longer. She wanted to die and kept asking me why she was alive, why the Lord wouldn't let her die. How do you answer a question like that? I had no idea.

This attitude seemed to prevail with my mother-in-law also. When Vern and I made the decision to put his mother into a nursing home, she almost begged for it. She seemed to have lost the energy to go to the dining room for her meals in her retirement home.

There were problems at the convalescent hospital -- her roommate being the biggest one -- but she didn't seem to resent being there. When we moved her in, she still was able to go to the dining room to eat with other residents. And she enjoyed going all over the home in her wheelchair.

Her neatest event was her daily visit to a man who had been her tablemate at the retirement home. She would go in and sit by his bed, holding his hand. It probably brightened both their days.

As she weakened, she ate in her room -- forgot where she was going when in her wheelchair -- thought the glasses on her stuffed bear were hers. However, with our regular visits and those of her granddaughter, she managed and so did we.

When you realize what is happening to an older relative it often is shocking. If you are the ones experiencing it while your siblings live far away, it is even harder. As explained earlier and will be discussed in Chapter Six, older people going through dementia of any type have many moments of lucidity. Too often the distant relatives who visit occasionally only see the good side. They do not experience the day-to-day problems that increase as the older person ages.

If you have a distant sibling, you may have the experience of your brother or sister coming to visit. At this moment, you watch your parent perk up and act perfectly normal, as if he or she has no problems at all.

This could be for any number of reasons. Your parent is happy to see his or her child and doesn't want that child to see anything is wrong. Or your parent is one of those people who simply loves company and won't let anything spoil the visit. Don't resent what is happening. However, take your sibling aside and tell what actually is going on with your parent. It is important for him or her to know the truth.

DD's parents lived in their own home over one hundred fifty miles from her. She didn't worry about them because her brother and sister-in-law were in the same town as the parents. They called DD with weekly reports including their mom's worsening condition when she was diagnosed with Alzheimers.

DD, her brother, and her sister-in-law, knew the caregiving strain would be too difficult for dad. "My brother and sister-in-law both were busy attorneys and couldn't monitor mom 24/7 if she and dad moved in with them," said DD. "They just could not take care of our parents."

The siblings had a sensible discussion and decided mom had to go to a nursing home. Three months after moving, mom died. Dad, who still was living in the family home, kept asking about going to visit his wife. The siblings told him that mom had died, but he refused to listen. A month after she died, he joined her.

Ailing older adults can stay positive in spite of illness and aging. Many older people who need care still keep a cheery personality, grateful for whatever help they get. Caregivers fortunate enough to care for these people tell me what a delight it was to have the opportunity.

> *One of my first husband's cousins willingly took her mother into her home when her mother became too frail to be alone. Her mother came from strong Dutch stock. All her life she kept an orderly home for her six children and husband. I'll never forget staying there and smelling the tantalizing baking odors in the morning. Hers was a strict Dutch Reformed religion which would not allow any cooking on Sunday. What wonderful foods were prepared on Saturday. And her house was always spotless.*
>
> *After the cousin's father died, the mother kept the house as long as her health allowed. Finally, the cousin took her mother to live with her family. "And mother never asked for anything," the cousin said. "I had a hard time even knowing when mother was ill because she never complained. I can truly say this caregiving experience was wonderful -- and I just hope I can be as wonderful."*

Necessary Duties

Finances and medications are the main items we need to be aware of and willing to help with as our loved ones declined in health. Older people think they still know how to maintain their financial transactions. However, and this is an increasing problem, telephone scammers are on the lookout for older people. And because so many older people have little social contact, they begin to talk to people (solicitors for example) who call on the phone. Soon they have been convinced it is all right to send money, or even give out social security numbers.

One friend was shocked to find her mother was writing checks to every solicitation by phone or mail. My friend tried to talk to her mother about this, but her mother would not listen. Finally, my friend had to take over her mother's checkbook, because that was the only way to stop these solicitations. By the way, her mother was writing large amounts on her checks and actually had no idea where the money was going.

Watch what checks are written and how the checks are written. Remember, even though I knew my husband's writing was becoming illegible, I didn't have the heart to tell him to stop writing checks. Thank goodness the bank teller told me the proper way to talk to my husband about his check writing and the resultant implications.

Even more frustrating are the medications. Personally, I feel doctors overmedicate -- but aside from that, older people do take a great many pills. And they forget either when to take the pills or end up taking too many. If your parents or any other older relative is still living in his or her own home, these medications must be monitored.

Almost everyone I interviewed said medications were a big concern for their loved ones. If a parent or parents were still living in their own homes, offspring were especially worried.

More than one person said they would go to their parents' home and discover full bottles of medication -- never touched because the parent "forgot to take the medicine."

In other cases, the older adult would think he or she had not taken the medicine and would take more than one dose each day.

This was a major reason parents were moved to a more secure environment -- either to their child's home or to a retirement or assisted living community.

These incidences must be included when you consider the next living arrangements for your loved ones. With this consideration comes the realization you now are acting the part of the parent. You are making the decisions. However, it's for the benefit of the person you have loved for years -- your opportunity to make a difference.

Who Are the Caregivers?

Throughout this chapter the implication has been that responsible caregivers generally are in their thirties or older. However, much credit needs to be given to those in their twenties, usually grandchildren, who also take on the caregiving role as best they can. Often, they are the most available people to care for a grandparent because parents are working, or even may be ill themselves. These young people take time from their own lives to help someone they love, and do it for no other reason than love and the realization they are the most logical people to help in this circumstance.

E's family had always been close. No gathering was complete without parents, grandparents, uncles, aunts, cousins. When E's grandmother was diagnosed with dementia there was no question about the family caring for her in her own home. However, the problem was everyone in the family had a job. They were able to afford care during the day, but nights were another matter.

Two grandchildren (siblings) immediately volunteered. The brother (B) would live in the home and do night duty, while the sister (E) took the three p.m. to nine p.m. shift. A registered aide (R. A.) would be there during the day -- seven a.m. to three p.m. E recently graduated from college and was starting a new job. She had looked forward to an apartment and socialization with friends. That was postponed and instead she lived with her parents as she took care of grandmother. She gave up most of her social life, with her parents occasionally stepping in for an evening.

"This was the right thing to do," said E. "The hardest part was trying to explain to my friends why I couldn't go to a party with them, or off on a long weekend. But I will always say it was the best thing I ever did in my life."

E said the hours of the care never actually ended. Sometimes she would get a call in the middle of the day, with grandmother asking, "Why aren't you here?" She said she felt guilty all the time she wasn't with her grandmother. While she liked and trusted the R.A.'s, they weren't family. "And family is what this is all about," said E.

The siblings became their own support group, often sitting together in the evenings to "de-compress." Both knew they could not have gone through those two years by themselves. Neither sibling wanted their grandmother in a nursing home, and their parents were far too busy professionally to be able to provide the care.

"Yes, there were bad days," said E. "Sometimes, I'd just go outside and scream. Then I'd remember grandmother. She was a tough lady -- she had to be, living on a ranch all her life. She cared for her husband when he got lung cancer, and she always was there for us.' Both siblings agree they have never regretted their two years "taking care of grandma."

Several families have had similar experiences. If the family has enough financial resources, they can opt to have 24/7 in-home care. Usually, a family member lives at the home as well, monitoring the care and being available for emergencies. This family member most likely is an unmarried son or daughter -- and occasionally a niece or nephew.

Another form of caregiving involves children or grandchildren who do it on a part time basis, or on call as needed. I earlier mentioned going to my mother's at night because I could not obtain nursing help. Children and grandchildren often give their weekends to the ill person, while working at a full time job during the week.

J had a different circumstance, this time with a step-grandmother. She had recently graduated from nursing school with a B. S. and gone to work in a hospital. She had her own apartment and lived over one hundred miles from her grandfather and his wife. However, when the wife became ill, J volunteered to go to her grandfather's each weekend to administer medicine and care for her step-grandmother. Again, hers was a close family and she never thought twice about giving this care.

"I was young and I had the experience to help," she later said. "This was my chance to give back what had been given to me."

Neither of the young women mentioned above questioned where their responsibilities lay. They were there to help, in this case with their grandparents who had been there for them when they were children. Now they were willing to serve in a new capacity.

Other members of the family also come to the aid of ill relatives when asked. Uncles, aunts, nephews, nieces all come to the aid of a loved one in times of need. This is part of the family unit, and while that unit may not be as strong as in the past, it still is a viable part of caregiving.

We have to realize as parents we served our children and now those children may be serving us.

Conclusion

None of us wants to see our relationship with our parents or grandparents change, but sometimes we have to become the parent instead of the child. We have to take over duties that are not always pleasant but necessary.

Decisions have to be made about where the loved one lives -- in his or her own home or a long term care facility or with a family member. This takes cooperation with everyone involved. Drivers licenses might have to be taken from the older person, a symbol of losing their independence.

Taking care of a family member in the home does not always have to be a burden, unless extreme dementia sets in. Many older people understand and try to be a "good guest." And many times grandchildren take on the responsibility of a grandparent.

The most difficult part of this process is realizing your parent might take on the role of the child. Patience and love will move everyone through this stage of caregiving.

CHAPTER FIVE

OVERCOMING THE JOURNEY'S ROADBLOCKS

Vern had COPD over ten years before his death. When he first had difficulty breathing at high altitudes or difficulty walking very far, I thought this would be the extent of his illness. But those of you who understand this disease know those are only the beginning steps.

We still were able to travel -- to Maui each year to visit his daughter, to Mexico where we stayed at a luxury resort and didn't do much traveling, on a cruise which is quite a confined area. In each place, I went to the beach to swim. He loved the beach but it was too far distant at the Mexican resort. On the cruise we were close to the outside doors so he didn't have far to walk to tour buses. He almost missed the penguins in Puerto Arenas, then decided to walk to them (and thus had irate bus passengers because it took him so long to return).

Two years before his death his disabilities increased. The trip to Yellowstone showed me his only recourse at this stage was oxygen and a method to get around. That was when I discovered that thinking you need something and actually getting it are two different things.

No journey is easy. The one upon which you are about to embark will probably be one of the hardest of your life (outside of raising your children!).

When I started my journey it was gradual. I didn't really think of what was happening until well into the process -- at which point

I knew this might be a long journey with many ups and downs. Take for example, my battle to get him oxygen.

While he had a hard time breathing, often gasping, his oxygen level was still too high according to Medicare standards. When he reached Stage 4 his pulmonary doctor recommended additional oxygen but had a difficult time getting it fulfilled. I overreacted when we met Vern's new case worker, yelling about the oxygen out of sheer frustration (and later apologizing to her because she was having as difficult time getting it as the doctor). It was my insistence and their perseverance that finally prevailed.

His doctor said, "Your husband now is in Stage 4 COPD. Let's make him as comfortable as possible."

With this comfort came the scooter he used both in and out of the house. This was a convenience that Vern enjoyed the rest of his life -- although with his increasing forgetfulness I had to be careful where he went.

I quickly became aware of his limitations, hence the need for new methods of care. Our RV resort in the Palm Springs area has an active group. One big attraction is taco night. Vern loved this time to eat and socialize. However, after trying to move him to a table, get his food and help him eat, I decided it was too difficult so stopped going. Fortunately, by this time he didn't recall that we went to Taco Night each month, making my decision much easier. I substituted a late afternoon dinner at our favorite Mexican restaurant.

Occasionally, he asked about going out to eat in restaurants. I could easily manage his entrance and exit at a few places -- especially if we went for a late lunch in the middle of the afternoon. But anything that was more difficult had me saying, "Oh, let's get take-out. It's more fun eating at home."

It probably wasn't more fun for him -- but it sure was for me. The eating arrangement he never objected to was during our trips. Lunch always was a picnic. I pulled off at a scenic spot where we could open our doors wide and relax with a view. This was better than a rest stop -- less noisy and he could take care of personal business.

This is the time to face one difficult problem, which was probably why I didn't enjoy going to eat or anywhere else -- bathrooms.

As Vern became increasingly weak, it was hard for him to walk all the way to the bathrooms -- whether a rest stop or a restaurant. At first, I went as far as the bathroom door and then he went in. However, sometimes he would stay and stay until I'd have to ask an entering man to see how he was. While restaurants weren't too bad, rest stops were terrible because the bathrooms were so far away.

I settled the problem two ways (until the end when I used diapers for a trip). Instead of rest stops, I'd go off a country road and find an isolated spot where he could relieve himself. In restaurants, I would have him use the handicapped restroom in the women's side -- always calling "man entering," or while in the stall and hearing someone entering "man inside." That worked so much better because I tired of men's restrooms.

Men in this situation with their wives also use women's restroom, calling out like I did.

Up until a year before his death Vern was able to take showers by himself. We have a large stall shower. Any hotel or condo which had a stall shower meant he also could use it himself. We had grab bars installed in our home shower (those really are handy for anyone). Also, I installed grab bars beside the toilet in two of our three bathrooms which helped him immensely. He could shower at the pool areas at our Palm Springs area place, making it easier for both of us. Pool showers were his area of shower choice for at least two years.

The idea of grab bar installation for both shower and toilet areas gave me peace of mind when Vern was alone. The man who installed the bars said they always could be removed if a new owner didn't like them. However, I find the shower bars convenient for me. I wish we had installed them sooner and would recommend this installation as soon as you decide to keep your loved one at home.

Even with the bars, I noticed Vern became more unsure of himself in the shower, very afraid of falling. Finally, I was helping him in and out of the shower and either washing him from the side or getting into the shower with him. I'm certain he enjoyed this a lot more than I did! Men caring for wives said in interviews they ended up with exactly the same shower arrangements.

> *Showering brought another interesting aspect to our lives. We had an active sexual life until his increasing weakness and illness. He still was interested in that aspect of our lives and couldn't understand my reluctance. He didn't stop to think of all I was doing with him toward the end -- very private matters that don't lend themselves to intimacy.*
>
> *This was probably one of the hardest parts of his life. I kept telling him that just holding me tightly in bed, just cuddling together was all that mattered. However, sex does remain a part of a great many lives right to the end.*

Friends undergoing many of the same things I have described say the incidents described above are huge roadblocks in the journey. Then they add some of the other roadblocks. Topping the list are spouses who become quite sarcastic, even cruel, when talking to their spouse. After the loved one has made a cruel comment, he or she cannot understand why their caregiver is angry or crying.

M is an only daughter. While she knows her brother loves their mother, she also knows he can't handle the increasing care load. Consequently, M agreed to the early care of her mother, who was in a retirement home, not nursing facility. Although her mother lived almost two hundred miles from M, she knew her mother had many friends in that vicinity, so moving her mother closer was not an option.

Mother was outgoing and loved by everyone at the retirement home. However, she became more and more confused, unable to handle her finances, and more demanding every time M visited.

When her mother broke her arm, M realized a skilled nursing facility was the next move. Her mother did not want to go but once she moved she immediately made friends with both staff and residents and was well liked. However, M also found her mother continually had a set of demands each time she visited. M had to buy extra food although food was provided at the facility. Her mother didn't like one care giver and demanded she be replaced. She wanted her room changed to one with more light. M calmly listened and tried to please her mother -- although she knew in reality nothing she could do would ever please her mother. M was cognizant that her mother had changed and just hoped she could keep her patience during this difficult time.

Caregivers also talk about the increasing demands of their spouse or parent. They agree that their loved ones probably don't even realize how demanding they have become. But as they are given additional care they begin to expect everything can be done for them. Keeping one's patience as a caregiver is very difficult at times like these.

In the final months family and friends told me I needed help with Vern. However, he did not want anyone else bathing or dressing him. Somehow, I couldn't confront his reluctant attitude.

Finally, with some persuasion on my part, he was willing to have someone come in for short periods while I either went to a business lunch or took my twin granddaughters somewhere. He trusted our housekeeper and allowed her to take care of him. Sometimes she and I would arrange it so he thought she was cleaning when in actuality she was taking care of him and feeding him lunch.

His case workers said there was Palliative Care (see Chapter Four) -- which I thought would be an excellent showering alternative. Vern reluctantly agreed on a male. By the time I had a name it was too late.

R and her husband have a caregiving business, going into it because they empathize and care about how older, ill people are treated. Their clients range from ones they see several times a week for small chores to people they care for eight hours a day a week or more at a time. But their shift does not stop at the end of the eight hours. They are available to each client on a twenty-four hour basis because they know many of their clients have no one else to call.

"We want our clients to know they have someone to depend on in a crisis," she said. Some clients have no family, so these professionals are the only ones to whom their clients can turn. Other clients have family, but those family members often are too busy to help their loved one. The professional fills that gap.

R and her husband also can fill in for the full-time unpaid caregiver who needs respite. "No one can go 24/7 forever," R said. "They need rest away from the situation. We know correct ways to bathe, dress and care for a client -- so no family member ever has to worry about our care."

This couple encouraged anyone in a caregiving situation to find additional professional help -- for both themselves and the patient.

The professional caregiver is there to fill a gap -- both for people who have no one to care for them and for unpaid caregivers who need respite. The rehabilitation and nursing facilities also fill a need, and sometimes are the only alternative for a family who has either health issues or work issues of their own.

The love and concern of professionals who enter caregiving at whatever level was emphasized when talking to Victor Reyes, Wagner Heights Nursing and Rehabilitation Center, Stockton, California. You must remember his words when considering the next moves for your loved one.

Reyes said that he learned how important his job and the jobs of all caregivers were when his mother had need of caregiving. "She was terrified of going to a nursing home," he said. That's when he realized the importance of being sure all employees first and foremost were caring individuals. "Not everyone can do the caregiving job," he continued. "It is a difficult one and not a job for money but for caring. It is a job from the heart and LOVE is all of it."

Many items need to be discussed months before your loved one's decline starts. Questions to be asked include: Are you going to be the only one caring for this individual? Is there anyone you can call if you need help? How would you contact a professional caregiver? Can your doctor help with this? When the decline starts it might be too late for these questions. All these concerns are roadblocks along this journey.

Not all caregivers have roadblocks along the journey. Some are very pleased with what happens because they can be there to help their loved one.

S was more than happy to care for her father when he came home with a terminal cancer diagnosis. He could not return to his house because his wife also was ill and couldn't cope with his fatal illness.

S and her husband took her father to their home and one or the other was with him constantly to the end. "My dad meant everything to me," S said. "I could always count on him for keeping our family together. Now it was my turn to be there for him."

When she brought him home he was happy just to be with her and her husband. She said when asked about going through caregiving: "Go for it. Don't be afraid. When it first comes and you think you can't do it, think again. It's the last thing you can do for your loved one before he or she leaves this earth. You'll be happy you could do this -- happy for the rest of your life."

Conclusion

No matter the journey, roadblocks usually occur. Among the first is the medical one. You are never certain proper medical care is being administered. When you see your loved one breathing heavily or perhaps not able to breathe correctly, you want to have relief for him or her, but don't know how to obtain it.

Be an advocate for your loved one. Read as much as you can and work closely with his or her physician to get the best care possible. Maintain charts and demonstrate you are well aware of what is happening. This type of persistence with Vern provided both oxygen and a scooter, helping both of us.

Know that your lifestyle will change. You may have to do "take out" rather than go to restaurants. You may have to determine what bathroom facilities you can use -- including using the handicapped restroom in the women's section which is more convenient for both sexes.

Bathing might become a real problem because your loved one no longer can get in and out of a tub. Perhaps he or she can't even be in the shower by themselves. Make plans. Add grab bars. And know you might be getting two showers a day!

Always remember -- your loved one's personality may change, either from medication or progression of a disease like Alzheimer's. Try to understand and keep your patience -- difficult but necessary. The roadblocks must be recognized, and then undertaken. You can do it.

CHAPTER SIX

A JOURNEY TO AGE RELATED DEMENTIA OR??

Vern's change occurred in late January 2010. Vern and I had gone to our place in the Palm Springs area to escape the cold weather in central California. We had a quiet, restful ten days as we prepared for my son, his wife, and two daughters to join us for a special visit.

By this time, I arose at least an hour before Vern, made the coffee, did my exercises and started to read the paper. He usually awoke about 8:30, ready for coffee and then breakfast. I heard him stirring in bed a little later than usual and went to see if I could help him.

He was babbling about his daughters -- pinpointing them at early ages. I tried to talk to him but he had only one thought. I asked him their ages and discovered he was at least forty years previous. I carefully talked to him about the girls, got him up and into the living room and poured his coffee.

His mind still was back in those previous days. By the time we finished breakfast I felt I must drive him home so the doctor could examine him the next day (Monday).

Packing the car was never easy but by twelve noon we were on the road and headed north. During that time he insisted that one of his old friends was driving us, and for a while he didn't know my name.

The next day we saw his doctor. Her diagnosis was "age related dementia."

This diagnosis of "age related dementia" often is first given to spouses and family when patients start the long road to decline. One feels that even doctors seem afraid to say the word Alzheimer's because of its fearful connotations. Yet as Vern's mental condition worsened along with his physical condition the totality of his illness should have been upper most in my mind.

Instead, I lived so much in the world of his deteriorating physical condition that I paid little attention to his mental condition. And the early signs of Alzheimer's can be so slight that Vern's getting lost occasionally or having difficulty forming words didn't seem that important.

Vern returned to his normal self after the initial diagnosis and for the next six months only had occasional lapses in memory. Then we took a two day mini trip to Northern California in July 2010. As we reached home he said, "That sure was nice of that man to help you drive home."

Enter a man visible only to Vern. This man was with us until Vern's death and often was joined by a woman visible only to Vern. Sometimes they even slept with us. He kept asking me their names and why they were with us. He also saw a dog, usually when we were eating, with the dog begging for scraps!

The most interesting thing about the woman was that Vern said he didn't really like her very much because she yelled at him. Usually, this happened after I had yelled at him about something -- and he projected my anger onto this woman.

His daughters called these people angels -- which could have been. I just became accustomed to them and went along with what was happening.

Vern had a case worker and a social worker from Kaiser for a year and a half. They had been assigned to his case because of his COPD. I had regular contact with both, discussing his latest COPD stages and asking advice about his sudden choking on food or his breathing difficulties. Although his mental condition worsened, I never thought to tell them of that dimension of his health because the physical was my main concern.

As I look back at his early dementia diagnosis, I wonder why no health professional suggested I read about dementia and Alzheimer's. If I had more information, I might have considered the seven stages: early, middle early, late early, early middle, middle middle, late middle and late or final. If I had examined these stages, I could have discussed them with the social or case worker. This could have given me a better grasp of what I was facing. He certainly moved from early to middle and late early during 2010.

T not only read about all the stages of Alzheimers as his wife progressed through them in a nearly ten year period, but worked out a chart about each one. Consequently, when he and his wife went for her check-ups he could hand the chart to the doctor to show her latest stage.

While this was an aid for the doctor, it actually was more of an aid to T. He knew by his wife's actions and symptoms the arrival of her next stage. He then was ready to face what was happening next, trying not to get discouraged but to cope with her ongoing illness.

Vern became paranoid, thinking I was having affairs with everyone from my handyman to a man who came to visit from the church. He could no longer write his name (the check writing earlier should have given me some clue) and certainly could no longer button a shirt (early middle stage). And then there was the anger and frustration, I think as much at his seeing the futility of his situation as anything else.

You've heard about the sudden bursts of anger with dementia patients. Vern had a sweet personality so when these bursts occurred -- and they were seldom- it totally surprised me. It depended on the day whether I would react or not -- and how tired I was. Fortunately, most times he blamed "that woman" for my angry outbursts! (A fascinating projection that saved me from his anger.)

Many caregivers told me that even as their spouses or parents declined mentally they remained quite sweet and docile. These patients are happy to go on walks each day, to sit in the park or along the river bank, to seemingly accept what is happening to them. Yet, at the same time they may suddenly see a futility in their lives and scream they wish they were dead or "Ah shit, what's happening?" This life change is not any easier for them than it is for the conscientious yet frustrated caregiver.

At no time did Vern's physician mention to me that his "age related dementia" seemed to be progressing. I had taken him in a year after his first diagnosis because of problems with incontinence. That was what she treated. I never thought to tell her of far more confusing events. If you even think there might be a chance of Alzheimer's, get all the information you can and then bring that information to the doctor. The physician needs to be aware of these changes. A later up-to-date diagnosis might have helped me deal better with what was happening.

Things became more and more confused for Vern in 2011. We could no longer go to the mountain cabin because of altitude and stairs. Stairs in the fifth wheel and out the door cancelled going to the trailer. However, it was cold at home in early January. So I mentioned going to our Palm Springs area place. Vern was excited and we went in late January.

He fell several times in our park model, sat only occasionally on the porch, and only went to the pool once because his physical limitations were too hard for me to manage.

On February 2, 2011 he fell in our living room. The man next door helped me put Vern to bed. Then he began to constantly babble about not being in bed, the room being totally messed up, and asking where our car was parked (he was looking for an antique truck he once owned). I realized he had gone over the edge and trying to put him in the car to take him home like the previous January would be impossible.

I called 911. He first went to emergency, then into the hospital.

Three days later a neurologist told me Vern had advanced Alzheimers. When I look back, I know he had changed considerably during that year but because he acted fairly normal when visiting his doctors I never asked for another evaluation.

The interesting part about this diagnosis was that I should have expected it. However, Vern's Alzheimer's was quite different from what I had read of other people. When we had a social visit with friends he usually could appear normal for an hour to an hour and a half. Then he would lapse into comments that were totally "off the wall" -- including seeing the dog or his male and female friend. Still, he never was completely into the stratosphere until that final night.

Another facet of Alzheimer's is the early age of some people's diagnoses. One caregiver told me his wife had first been diagnosed at fifty seven years old. During her early years she still tried to work, until she realized her confusion at even small jobs. He spent the last six years of her life as a caregiver, still trying to travel with her and lead as normal a life as possible. They were able to do this until the final six months of her life -- but even then the caregiving burden never left this man's mind because he kept her at home the entire time.

Children of parents diagnosed with Alzheimer's face major hurdles. As they learn the stages of the disease they know their parent can no longer live alone -- or that the parent has become a burden to a spouse. These children are faced with a dilemma. They are convinced their mother or father can no longer take care of the spouse. Now they have to go to a parent and convince that parent it would be better to put the other parent in assisted living or a nursing home. If a parent lives alone, the children with the help of the parent's physician must move the parent to a facility. Approaching their parent is the most difficult part of this procedure.

When you are ready to move a parent to a facility, obtain lists of all possible choices. If the parent still is mobile, can feed and dress himself or herself, there are assisted living facilities that give more freedom. If the parent has digressed to the point where he or she needs dressing and feeding, nursing homes are available. Visit each one before you make your final decision.

K was an active man and full of a bubbling personality. Suddenly, he started falling. In his early seventies, he was still robust and much too heavy for his wife to lift. The wife and daughters took him to a clinic for evaluation and this time heard a "vascular dementia" diagnosis. The three woman thought they could deal with this and brought him home. But when he continued to fall and was more and more confused, the daughters knew this burden was too difficult for their mother. At first, his wife resisted the idea of moving him to a care facility. Then, as she became more exhausted, realized it was the only solution. Now wife is more rested and he happily goes along with what has happened. Better for all.

One interviewee talked about how her mother with Alzheimer's was living with her brother and his wife who both worked. When the mother began to regress, they realized they couldn't watch her 24/7 and agreed to move her to assisted living.

"It was none too soon," said the interviewee. "Mom went from the sedate woman we knew to stripping off her clothes or trying to escape the facility. This was the best move we made."

Another interviewee talked of her mother moving into the assisted living facility and suddenly refusing to get out of bed. "She just laid there and mumbled and mumbled. We realized the necessity of the home -- but hated to see what had happened."

When Vern's final diagnosis came -- after all those years of doubt on my part -- he was fortunate to drift into a state where he was comfortable. I did feel he knew what was happening, even if he couldn't express himself. As his children and grandchildren visited, as my daughter-in-law talked to him about the Bible, I noticed a relaxation. He knew where he would go next, but waited for his youngest daughter to come from Hawaii. Shortly after she arrived to be with him, he moved to the next life.

When a neighbor in Palm Springs heard about Vern's Alzheimers diagnosis, she told me about her brother-in-law who fell and quickly regressed into Alzheimers. She finished by saying, "He only lasted three weeks. It was that quick -- from the diagnosis to his death." That was the time frame for Vern, also.

Conclusion

The diagnosis of age related dementia should be a sign for spouses and relatives to know their loved one may be nearing another phase and the start of Alzheimer's. It is important to know the stages of Alzheimer's and to face the fact that a loved one will continue to decline.

This means talking openly with the doctor about what is happening to the patient, not only in the physical realm but the mental one. Avoiding this does not change the diagnosis. Thought needs to be given about the next move for the patient. Where is the best placement for the patient? Can the caregiver provide all the necessary care? And can the caregiver survive under the increased pressure?

Age related dementia and Alzheimer's are never easy on anyone -- but especially hard on the caregiver. Give careful consideration to each step in the process -- and if necessary be willing to turn care over to an assisted living or skilled nursing facility.

This move will be beneficial to all concerned.

CHAPTER SEVEN

SHOULDA/COULDA AIDS FOR THE JOURNEY

As I look back on the final three years of Vern's long illness, I realize he enjoyed a life of going and doing. Friends later commented that we still traveled and did so many different things that he obviously didn't want to die. Could be...

People accuse me of being a "wandering soul" and perhaps that is true. I own a time share and always have looked for the bargains associated with it -- inexpensive condo vacations. Consequently, during those final three years we went to the Southern California coast a few times, out to the desert and to Sedona and Tucson, Arizona, plus the trips to Branson and Yellowstone. In addition, we could go to our Palm Springs area place, to our trailer near the Monterey coast, and to our place in the mountains. Yes, I guess it did look like constant movement.

Vern loved everywhere we went -- and while the packing and unpacking of the car often was a strain, I knew he was happy. His happiness helped me to cope with his steady decline.

This chapter is essential to read right after you start your journey. I wish I'd thought of or been told about some of these ideas early on. Too often, once your journey begins, and certainly during it, you are faced with so many new routines you become overwhelmed. Those extra duties mean you never think of other ways to make your loved one's journey more pleasant.

Unfortunately for Vern, most of these ideas came to me after he died. As I was cleaning our house in preparation for sale (something I had wanted to do earlier but knew with his condition I could not), I noticed several ways I could have kept him entertained.

He was provided with one entertainment -- his talking books. These were sent because of his failing eyesight. If you have a loved one with failing eyesight, get confirmation from their ophthalmologist and then contact the National Center for the Blind. These books are free and sent by mail through a program operated by the National Library of Congress.

Almost every day when we were at home, I'd put one of his books on the tape recorder. Sometimes he would listen and sometimes fall asleep. He was alert enough not to like modern books with swearing, sex and violence. However, he loved Westerns and books of that genre -- so those kept him involved while I cleaned, did other duties, or wrote.

However, I totally goofed in one area and could have done so much more. When I opened cupboards to start my clean-up packing, photo albums and family and trip videos cluttered the shelves. Right away I knew what I should have done throughout his illness.

Although his eyes were dimming, he still could have enjoyed looking at those pictures -- both our trips and families. We could have sat and talked about those good times, recalling with humor much of what had happened to us -- the fun and also the occasional disaster. He could remember, perhaps more of the past than the present, and these could have made a pleasant day for him. If I put him in a brighter light he could view the pictures by himself. Why didn't I think of that when he was alive?

This leads me to the other shoulda/coulda -- all our videos of trips and families. We had enough to keep him entertained for weeks. He was so proud of his videos, took them constantly on our trips and cruises. In fact, he always laughed when he saw my video of the St. Petersburg (Leningrad in those days) port which we were told couldn't be recorded. I'm sure he would have enjoyed seeing them again and again. In fact, with his failing memory he probably wouldn't even have remembered that he had seen that video two weeks previously. And to see the family members ten and twenty years previously could have jogged more important memories.

One more memory booster I discovered were tapes he had recorded years previously when his family was young. I didn't realize we had those around and know he would have loved to hear his daughters, his first wife and all his relatives and friends talking to him. However, he had packed these items away in a suitcase and I didn't find them until it was too late.

These are examples of things that can keep your loved one entertained as well as remembering the past.

And don't forget about humor. A study which had Alzheimer's nursing home residents actively participate in a weekly clowning session proved therapeutic. The session had music, mime, and humorous props to get them involved. At the end of the session and during the next week they were less agitated.

Think about ways you can implement this in your own home. It probably also would be good for you, the caregiver. I know I always tried to add some humor to our lives, especially at meals and bedtime. And Vern always laughed with me.

Important Visits

Another shoulda/coulda involves people I needed to ask over for an hour long coffee or tea break. I say hour because it usually was that length of time Vern could stay focused with visitors. In an earlier chapter I talked about inviting people to come over, but it always was in a casual way. Most friends just won't take you up on the invitation, either because they do not want to intrude on you, or really don't enjoy visiting sick people. When they are specifically invited, however, they will make the effort.

Vern always enjoyed the visits, although by the end of the hour he sometimes was in a different place than the rest of us. Later, I was talking to some close friends who visited regularly and they said his "zoning" out was expected and didn't bother them at all.

Any visit that bolsters the patient's ego is an important visit which needs to be cultivated.

Several interviewees voiced the same comment about having friends visit. They emphasized that the visits didn't have to be long -- just friendly. One woman who took care of her father during his final days, mentioned the big smile across his face when a friend arrived to visit him.

"He might not even have remembered who the person was, but the idea that someone cared to come and talk with him made a big difference," she said.

Another woman talked about church visitors who came to get information about Christian living. Her father had been quite involved with the church and often helped newcomers come to know the Lord. When her father was asked to help anyone with their faith he was more than willing to cooperate. He felt like he could help on the path to salvation, which made him extra happy at this stage of his life.

End-of-Life Decisions

While this may seem a strange place to put end of life decisions, this is actually a "shoulda/coulda" you need to think of early. Three areas are important: living will to explain end-of-life desires, funeral arrangements, and possible plans for the time immediately before the end-of-life period. I've already done the first two for myself. In Vern's case, he had signed his end-of-life wishes, which also was required by Kaiser. This had been done by both of us shortly after we married so none of our children had to face that decision. He postponed making funeral arrangements until a friend experienced a cremation problem for her deceased brother. When Vern heard the complications, he agreed to sign all the papers for his funeral arrangements. This happened in

December 2010. However, neither of us thought about possible plans for the time immediately before the end of life.

You may have one more decision to make if your loved one does not have a living will. W and her siblings had a critical decision to make about their mother after she was placed in assisted living. Their mother refused to eat. At this point, the doctor and nursing home suggested a food tube. They had never been in a situation like this, so agreed to the tube.

W says: "We should have just let her go, but the nursing home put us on a guilt trip -- mom had only been in there a few months and we were still feeling guilty (about putting her there). If we had to do it over, we wouldn't have let the home talk us into it. They have everything to gain by doing this -- another breathing body paying monthly fees. It's not like this was a temporary thing. It wasn't like she had a condition from which she would recover and not need the feeding tube any more."

W and her siblings still are upset by how guilty the nursing home made them feel.

Never be pressured into something you may not feel is right. In other words, research all the types of things you may face at the end of your loved one's life, and especially at the very beginning of a terminal illness. Be sure you and your siblings agree on the next steps and stand by what you've agreed on. You never should feel guilty about your decisions.

Both of us were like many of you when it came to end-of-life plans beside the medical. You just expect to die -- hopefully right in your home. My father and mother both died suddenly in their homes as did my first husband. Vern's first wife, his father, and his mother were in the hospital when they died, and family was with them. Many people dying of a terminal illness spend their last days in their own homes surrounded by family; others in the hospital. The family has a choice. Make sure you choose one you'll be most comfortable with.

In the final phases of many illnesses, your loved one is offered the option of Hospice. That's an excellent option because it is an awesome opportunity to see caring people in action.

J saw Hospice in action the final days of her husband's life and was grateful he could stay in their home. She had been through a year of trial with her husband, and knew he would not want to go to the hospital.

Their trial started when he had lung surgery in July 2008. During surgery, the doctor cut a nerve on her husband's right side. From that time on, her husband always was in pain.

But he never complained, having a high tolerance for pain. However, now he needed oxygen and couldn't be involved in all his normal activities.

By May 2009, they were told he could have Hospice. That's when he said, "Just as long as I don't have to leave my home. I want to celebrate my birthday here."

Celebrate he did with his entire family with him in his house. He died later in May.

J says she'll always remember her husband's strength and how he wanted to do things for himself, right up to the end.

Hospice comes into your home to make both the patient and the caregiver more comfortable. Usually, a hospital bed also is brought in for the comfort of the patient.

However, Hospice also comes into the hospital or assisted living in the final days. If your loved one is in a hospital, or assisted or skilled nursing facility you must consider this fact -- when he or she goes on Hospice they become a private care patient. This is a good time to decide whether you might want to take them home (if it is possible) so they can spend their last days or hours in familiar surroundings. Unfortunately, this was an option I had not considered.

You must think about the final days very carefully. I wish I had, but never knew I would be in this type of circumstance. This is very important to think about now -- probably one of the most important decisions you will make. If the doctor tells you that your loved one has a limited time (which never was quite conveyed to me until the last two days), you might want to take him or her home for that final rest before death.

How Vern would have loved to be in his own bed at the end. He wasn't eating at all and had 24/7 oxygen so all I would have had to do is his simple hygiene. My daughter-in-law is a nurse, so she could have administered the morphine. And we would have had plenty of family help at that point -- like 24/7. While we were allowed into the nursing facility twenty-four hours a day, it just wasn't the same as it would have been if he was at home.

I didn't know all this. Transporting him home would have been expensive but it would have been worth it for his end of life. THINK ABOUT THIS.

Caring for Yourself

One final note in this shoulda/coulda chapter -- think about yourself. Several books have been written with warnings for caregivers (see the bibliography at the end). All have good advice, especially about coping skills and handling your emotions. From these come excellent points like these:

- Pace yourself
- Learn to say "no"
- Go with the flow
- Stop and think about yourself once in a while

I know these sound logical, but the pace often becomes so rapid you never get the chance to think about yourself. You may find yourself very angry -- several interviewees have told me that. You are angry about the entire situation and probably at your loved one for putting you into this situation (although you don't want to admit those feelings). Maybe you're even angry at yourself for getting to this place in your life. Accept -- blow off steam -- and keep on going, but now use the above suggestions.

Looking back, there were many shoulda/coulda points I needed to make and didn't. May this help you not to make the same mistakes -- it will make the journey easier.

Conclusion

When you are finished with this journey you may look back on several "shoulda/coulda things you could have done for your loved one. While you may be taking him or her out as much as possible, and they enjoy it, you can do other things right at home. Look for your photo albums, videos and even recorded tapes. Give your loved one the album, and give yourself a rest by going through it with him or her. Put on the videos, both of family events and trips. And if you have recorded tapes of the family, play those and listen for enjoyment. These photos, videos and tapes will bring unexpected happiness to your loved one.

Visits by family and friends are very important both for you and your loved one. You may have to issue the invitations because often people don't realize your need for outside visits. They might think you are too busy and don't want to interfere. Assure everyone that a visit is perfect, even if they have to be the entertainment!

Make end-of-life decisions BEFORE the final stage of your loved one's life. You can do this through living wills, pre-planned funeral arrangements, and deciding where your loved one wants to be at the end of life -- home or hospital.

Don't let the "should/couldas" slip by you.

CHAPTER EIGHT

NEVER STOPPING IN THE JOURNEY

Journey is the name of this book for a specific reason. Vern and I started our marriage with a series of trips domestically and overseas, bought a fifth wheel so we could travel more, and never stopped during the entire duration. Even as Vern became weaker, he still thought going on any type of trip would be wonderful -- and continuing to travel is what we did during those last three years.

It helped that we had many places to go to, plus the convenience of the timeshares we could use through two companies to which we belonged. I tried to find as many weeks as possible -- to the Southern California beaches, to the Arizona desert and a day or two in San Francisco. These gave him a change of scenery -- and let's face it, gave me that same change even if I had to load and unload all his equipment each time.

The trips to our places usually were for a day or two. The altitude at our mountain house bothered him if we stayed too long. He did love sitting on the deck and watching the birds and squirrels. The fifth wheel trailer became more difficult for him to manage because of the inside stairs, but we still tried to get in one or two nights.

The Palm Springs area place was a longer time because of the distance. He sat on our porch and waved to passersby or dozed in the warm sunshine. I can honestly say I'm glad I never stopped our trips -- for both of us.

While the title of this chapter may sound strange, I think never stopping is a big part of our journey through the caregiving process. I've talked to several people about the book's title and some rebel at the word "duty."

"How can you even call it a duty? Like something that HAS to be performed?" Several have said. "You were doing an act of love."

Yes, this caregiving process was done in love, but as the time progressed, duty also entered the picture. After all, one day follows the other with a routine that becomes so common place it almost is done by rote.

Other people I interviewed said they totally agreed. The 24/7 grind is just that -- something that takes over one's life. (One person said it is more like twenty-seven or thirty hours a day.) As a caregiver, you know you have to do certain things each day -- changing bed linens AGAIN or washing one more load of clothes, or driving to another doctor's appointment, plus many extra chores. You also know if you don't do those things, no one else will do them -- hence the word duty.

N, a professional man, commented that unless someone has already experienced caregiving no one would realize the collateral damage being done to the caregiver.

He described his step-father who was caring for his mother. She had lapsed into Alzheimers. His step-father became quite tired, to the point where N and his three brothers knew something had to be done. The four sons went to the step-father to plead with him to get help. "It was interesting that it was the four stepsons, not his own children, who realized what was happening," he said. "I guess it was because we four saw mom more and knew what all this extra care was doing to our step-father. We understood what was happening to him."

They finally convinced the step-father to get help.

While you may become demoralized by all that is happening, you can do some things both for yourself and your loved one -- not necessarily easy things, but things that can help you through the day. Our day together started with his cup of coffee, and me reading him the comics -- his favorite page of the paper. After breakfast we read and talked about the daily lesson in our Bible booklets. This gave him a good time to reminisce. If he didn't feel like dressing, I'd take him out on the deck (if warm) or over to his big chair by the fire. He didn't like TV but did enjoy his books on tape. His listening to the books gave me time to clean up, wash clothes, etc. Those morning routines also helped me to focus on the rest of the day.

Each caregiver has his or her own routines -- ones that help the loved one and the caregiver. And each caregiver finds ways to make the time more pleasant for both of them.

S's father came to live with her and her husband two years after her mother died. He had a forty acre ranch and soon realized he was unable to continue to work it. With reluctance, he agreed to live with S and her husband. "I don't know about him," S said, "but it was the best decision I ever made. It was a most gratifying time because I had a chance to learn about him and his life. We'd talk about events both in his life and when I was small. Both of us looked forward to these times -- a special part of the day."

After S retired, she bought a computer, thinking she'd learn all about it. But she found a better place to spend her day -- talking with her father. Her father also enjoyed going out in the car -- never rejected a trip although his aches and pains had become more intense.

He was with S for six years. The first years he used a walker but as his strength declined, he had a wheel chair. She said throughout his illness he was a gentle person, good spirited, and never complaining. He went to church until he became too weak, then listened to the sermons on a cassette.

S's final comment, "I knew my dad as a young man, but never really knew him. Caregiving time opened a window for me. It was a treasured time."

Facing Difficult Times

As mentioned previously, Vern loved to go places in the car -- anywhere including a short jaunt to the post office. He just liked getting out of the house.

It wasn't always the easiest thing to get him into and out of the car. While our convenient Chevrolet HHR held everything I needed to take -- his scooter, oxygen, mister, walker, etc -- it was small and sometimes difficult for him to enter. That didn't bother him because he was going someplace. Fortunately, I had great health so I could manage all the challenges.

After Vern's death, someone asked me if I was ever able to go to the store during my 24/7 care. "Of course," I'd say. "Vern was up to going to the store or on any other errands whenever I was ready."

He didn't mind sitting in the car. Many times when he was still lucid he watched people -- a perfect past time for anyone. Other times he would sleep. Somehow, I never worried about him alone in the car -- both because we were in safe places the majority of the time, and I simply trusted nothing would happen. I didn't allow fear to ever enter my consciousness. I had enough other things to worry about!

We did travel back and forth to our many places until the last few months. I learned to go in many types of bathrooms -- a real necessity. At first, I would try to let him go in -- but when I had to send men in to see how he was doing I decided there were more practical ways.

For one thing -- rest stops often have bathrooms too far from the car. He was exhausted by the time he finally got to one. I learned about the truck stops or gasoline stations which had closer bathrooms as well as handicapped bathrooms for both sexes.

At first, I would try to take him into the men's bathroom (after checking it out) because there always is at least one stall. However, this became tedious -- so used the women's handicapped stall, as explained earlier.

The reality is that bathrooms are something we all have to face if we take our loved one on a jaunt -- until they are in protective underwear. Many times I'd park on a lonely road both to eat lunch and so he could relieve himself. This is logical for a man but not quite the logical way for those of you with females.

Vern loved to eat out, which we did until the very end. I tried to arrange our meals so they were in the middle of the afternoon. This was done for two reasons: (1) We could skip lunch and have an early dinner and (2) there weren't as many people in the restaurant at that time of day. Our meals were in casual places -- Denny's, IHOP, Chili's, Marie Callender's, or our favorite Mexican restaurants -- places with easy parking and nearby tables. Tables, not booths, were my choice because they were much easier to use with his walker.

Toward the end we had to rely on take-out. I just didn't have the energy any longer to maneuver him into the restaurant. Before this happened, we occasionally went to the Casino buffets. Valets were eager to get a wheelchair for him. I had to pick out all his food but he was familiar enough with these places to make it easier on both of us. And once in a while I loved treating myself to a shrimp buffet.

I guess much of what I am writing is like a story I read in trusting in a Supreme Being. I trusted that we would make it -- that each and every time I went out with Vern he and I could manage.

I like that story because it talks about trust being like driving a car at night. Our headlights never shine all the way to our destination; they just illuminate about one hundred sixty feet ahead. But we trust those headlights because all we really need is enough light to keep going forward.

And what I needed was just enough trust to know that we would make it wherever we were. Also, it seemed people were always available when I needed them -- helping him from the table or opening a door. Actually, they seemed to appear more as he became more frail.

Throughout this entire procedure I tried to keep myself and my mind busy. My favorite project was deciding to look for different things to do, things I hadn't done in a while. Reading books I had bought but never had a chance to read. Writing my book ideas, helped along by my publisher. Watching some new TV show, which Vern also could enjoy. Finding old movies we'd enjoyed previously and could watch again (he never remembered them anyway).

He loved shows on Discovery Channel where people were doing odd or dangerous jobs. I think he saw these shows as examples of what he once did when he ran his crane. These were the things he still enjoyed and I wanted him to stay involved.

I managed to be amused at these little things. I think he did, too. I am certain we can always learn new things, even in a time of strife like extensive caregiving. Also, keep in mind the idea we are being transformed -- learning that whatever happens we can survive.

Although you're now involved in constant routine, you can't stop doing it. Your loved one needs you. You often will become exhausted but you have to realize you are accomplishing a new pattern. You are giving of yourself, and someday you can step back to evaluate your successes and your failures during this time. Never feel guilty at that time because you truly have done all you could to make the last days of your loved one's life happy.

And as mentioned previously, bring in family and friends as often as you feel comfortable. Let them know not to expect you to entertain with hot coffee and cookies, but rather that they are the entertainers with love and stories. Let them know they are bringing joy to you and your loved one.

Stopping? No. Caring and moving on as best you can because you have been placed in a special place at a pivotal time in your life.

F and her husband have a most inspiring caregiving story -- that of devotion of a child and her husband to a mother -- always done in love and caring.

F and her husband didn't have any children during their long marriage. "And maybe there was a reason for that," said F.

F's mother was an active woman at seventy-one years old, still working in a department store part time. Her mother had high blood pressure and treated it regularly with medication. When she moved some furniture and had some upper arm and chest pain she didn't think anything of it.

Mother joined F and her husband on a road trip from California to Wyoming to attend a graduation. On their way, they stopped overnight in Wendover, Nevada and there mother's pain resumed. Quickly, they drove her to the nearest city -- Salt Lake City. What started as a heart attack, moved to a stroke.

Mother ended in a deep coma the first month after her stroke. After staying in Salt Lake City for almost two months, F and her sister decided mother needed to be near them so medi-vacced her to Stockton, their hometown, although she still was in a coma. After almost two months, mother came out of her coma but still needed almost four years of rehabilitation.

Then came decisions. F's sister could not take care of their mother. F and her husband, although in Southern California, decided they would redo their home to accommodate mother.

They picked her up and drove her down -- to stay with them for the rest of her life.

"We never regretted what we did," said F. "We tried to give her as much of a life as we could. She was in a wheelchair, but that didn't stop us from taking her out to eat or to the movies. She always enjoyed going with us."

Mother had several mini-strokes and went to the hospital two times for congestive heart failure. That was when mother begged them not to let her go back again to the hospital. F and her sister agreed. Sister came to help and Hospice was at hand.

"She died at our home," F concluded. "Caring for her was the natural thing to do -- she was my mother."

Conclusion

Never stopping during this journey is good for you and your loved one, if you have the stamina to do it.

Find places you can visit, if possible. These probably should be near your residence, unless you have another home. Plan carefully when you go, pack a lunch, and take rest stops for both of you.

When it becomes too difficult to take your loved one places, invite friends to visit. Remind them, they might be the entertainers rather than the entertained. Have family visit often so they can talk of the "old days."

Never stop the journey. It's better for you and your loved one.

CHAPTER NINE

THE JOURNEY ENDS -- OUT OF THE DARKNESS

A uthor's Note: I'm writing this chapter almost four months after my husband's death. Once again, I've come to our place in the Palm Springs area, this time to close it for the summer (temperatures are just now moving toward the hundreds). I've just been to the pool and after swimming my laps, sitting and reading a Dean Koontz' novel, *The Door to December*. The psychiatrist/mother has started therapy to bring her daughter back to normality. I am a family counselor without the necessary hours to become a therapist but I understand methods to bring people back to whatever it is we call reality and normality. I thought of the last year with my husband and how I could never sit and read at the pool. If he was with me on his scooter I always had to worry about what he would do next. And if I left him at our small place for a half hour or so, I always had to hurry back to be sure he was all right. Now, I have that time and as I went to take a shower the light dawned for me -- after four months I am moving out of a darkness that started almost four years previously.

Those of you reading this book and this final chapter, and also serving as caregivers may not think you are in any type of darkness. You think of yourselves as nurturing, caring individuals who are doing everything you can for your loved one while still leading life as you want it.

Whatever you are thinking -- don't be fooled. For however many years you have been performing caregiving tasks, your life has been anything but normal. There is only one goal for you each day -- to be sure the one for whom you are caregiving is having a good day. For many of you, especially those with no help, your day starts as soon as your loved one awakens. Maybe you have to take him or her to the bathroom. You put on his or her slippers, maybe a bathrobe, and help the person to the kitchen table or living room for that first cup of coffee.

And the day progresses from there. Eating breakfast and perhaps helping to feed your loved one. Maybe a shower or a sponge bath and then dressing him or her. You try to make your loved one feel like he or she is making choices -- taking out a shirt and saying would you like to wear this one? An affirmative smile is always nice.

Then it's to a favorite chair to watch TV or listen to a book. Maybe you read the comics to him or her, or some of the newspaper headlines.

Time for yourself? Sure, when you clean up the breakfast dishes, or wash clothes, or straighten out the bed. If you're like me, you try to find some time at the computer -- or pulling weeds, or watering -- but always in the back of your mind is checking on your loved one to be sure he or she is all right.

In my case, my husband loved to go driving with me, so no matter where I was going -- grocery shopping or to get my hair cut, he went along. He didn't get out of the car (I knew he couldn't get out when I left him because I always had to help him in and out of the car). He was perfectly happy just sitting there.

When he became sick enough to be in the hospital and later skilled nursing (only nineteen days from start to finish), I was at the facilities at least eight to ten hours a day. By the time I arrived home I was so tired I could barely fix some dinner and fall into a restless sleep.

And that restless sleep continued for at least two months after he died. I told myself once I was through with his death, the celebration of life and the children visits, that I could resume my normal life. Consequently, people would ask me how I was doing and I'd say, "Just fine. Now I have only myself to think of." In part that was true because I had been through so much during those three plus years.

It was wonderful to go to lunch with friends I hadn't seen in years. I could go places with my grandchildren without worrying about my husband. I still fixed nourishing meals for myself which also lasted two or three days! Slowly, I began to regain the fifteen pounds I had lost.

Yet, my life wasn't really normal. We had too many residences. I was sure I had to go to each of them regularly, which meant I was always on the road. I still had obligations because of my writing, so tried to fit in those. I decided to sell one house and had to clean it up. (NOTE: If yours is a first experience with a death of a loved one, don't rush into any major decisions like house selling for a least a year. Remember, mine was a second death and I had been thinking about what I would do with the house when that death came.)

Cleaning up to move meant a storage unit while I figured out what to do with all my stuff. It also meant a yard sale to eliminate much of my clutter. Consequently, I never slowed down -- up early, to bed late -- working on cleaning the house, weeding the yard, cleaning my swimming pool, and driving here and there to other houses.

The one good thing was a book originally scheduled for October 2010 publication that was moved to June 2011 publication and then to July 2011. That was perfect. My husband was too ill for me to do any PR in October, and I really wasn't fit for June either. By July I finally had come out of the darkness and was ready for new challenges -- and the book PR.

When my husband was ill I told myself that when my caregiving was over I'd need at least four to six months of a reflective "away period" to regain my perspective. But my first four months didn't give me time for that -- until that revelation at the pool in Palm Springs. When that happened I felt like everything had fallen away. Yes, I still had obligations -- but I could now go ahead and fulfill them at my own pace, not someone else's. I could start to relax and decide what I'd want to do with "the rest of my life!"

One more thing -- about six months before my husband died I suddenly realized my spiritual side was not being fulfilled. I was doing chores morning to night, and while we were reading spiritual resources daily I wasn't giving more time to a spirituality I had throughout my life. I found some books I loved and began reading them again (hadn't done it through much of our marriage). I had to take time for myself. When Vern died those books became a daily morning habit -- taking me through the days and helping me to "take one day at a time" (as the song goes).

This entire chapter is written to show you that you also will someday be out of the darkness and into a new light. Yes, you miss your loved one. Yes, now you think of the many other things you could have done for him or her. Yes, many of you wonder how you will go on.

You have been through a great deal. This book was written to show you how to deal with much of it when your loved one is with you -- hopefully giving you fewer regrets when he or she is gone.

Now is your time -- to do what you want or what you feel you missed -- to travel, to volunteer, to spend more time with grandchildren or children or friends.Remember those ancient words, "There is a time . . ."[1]

This is your time -- out of the darkness. A new journey begins.

---

1. Ecclesiastes 3:1

POST NOTE:

NO GUILT AT JOURNEY'S END

Remember the woman who said she was so relieved when her mother (who she took care of for years) died, and then she quickly added that she felt so guilty for feeling that way?

Guilt has a tendency to follow us, if we allow it. We've just spent anywhere from one to several years caring for a loved one and suddenly we no longer have that responsibility. We feel so relieved to get on with our own lives -- to live each day without that daunting routine.

Then we begin to think of what we could have done to make the journey easier for our loved one -- forgetting how tired we were or all the circumstances involved. Those "shoulda/couldas" discussed in Chapter Seven begin to envelop us.

We could have taken him or her home from the nursing home when Hospice arrived. We could have visited even more when the loved one was in a nursing home. We could have.... Well, you know how the couldas add up.

One woman took care of an uncle who was in his early hundreds. She agreed with the family that she wanted to do it and took excellent care of her beloved uncle. As he declined, he ended up with Hospice. Because this woman was a nurse, Hospice told her she could administer his morphine. Consequently, they left her uncle's care in her hands -- rarely coming to the house.

Of course, the uncle declined and the pain was worse and she administered more morphine. He died at 102 years old.

Now the woman blamed herself for his death -- that perhaps she had given him too much morphine. Her guilt piled on after his death to the point where she could barely function.

The man described above led a good life and led it far longer than most people. This woman did all she could for him. There is absolutely no reason to have guilt at this point.

Death comes to all of us -- that's the deal we made when we were born. Fortunately, most of us live a long time -- but not all. We have to enjoy each day but we can't feel guilty about something that has passed.

When your loved one dies, keep the thought that you did everything you could for him or her. If you have any type of faith at all, you now know that your loved one is in a better place, experiencing whatever is the next journey.

Take a big sigh and move on with your life -- showing that your actions are an example of your strength in what you have been through. That's life -- the end of one journey and the beginning of another.

If you simply believe that death is the final step of life, then you must accept this finality while at the same time keeping all of your memories of a special life with your loved one.

AUTHOR'S THOUGHTS ON:

Faith -- Each of us is on our own path in life with many of us believing in a spiritual side while others believe only in our humanity. As you have gathered while reading this book, mine is a belief in the spiritual. Without my strong faith in a Supreme Being (God in my case) becoming a 24/7 caregiver would have been extremely difficult. In fact, I don't think I could have survived.

There never was a time in my life when I didn't believe ina God or a Supreme Being or whatever the title. Although I didn't go to church often as a child and we never said grace at meals, I still believed in a strong Being somewhere above and around me.

I prayed often -- first for my husband and then to give me patience. I can think of countless times when those prayers revealed a new perspective or a chance to relax for an hour or two, or just a feeling of someone taking my hand.

For those of you who believe, **REMEMBER** faith is a big component of keeping you sane during the caregiving period.

Death -- My life was filled with early deaths which is why I have never feared death or found it anything more than the next phase of life itself. As I explained earlier, my parents died young as did my first husband. And in-between were the grandparents, aunts, and uncles. The first death I remember was a former student of my dad's who was killed shortly after the U. S. entered World War II (I was probably six or seven at that time). That's when I heard about heaven and life after this one.

I have no idea where I will be going after this life or if I will see any of my loved ones -- but whatever happens -- death is just another step in the long progression. Therefore, with all my husband's suffering, I felt he was finally released to a new beginning when he died.

Resources

My greatest resources were the wonderful people I interviewed throughout the United States. I used letters for their names for two reasons. First many opened up and said honestly how they felt about the entire caregiving episode, and I felt these were private thoughts to me. Secondly, there were times when I combined two similar experiences into one story. So, if you are reading and say, "Wait a minute. That's not quite what I said." Don't worry. You've just been combined!

And special thanks to the people who worked with Vern and I during his illness: Victor Reyes, admissions coordinator, Wagner Heights Rehabilitation and Nursing Facility, Stockton, California; Denita Davis, Social worker, Kaiser Permanente, Stockton, California; Christie Milhaus, case worker, Kaiser Permanente, Stockton, California; Dr. Twana Adeshina, (Vern's personal physician), Kaiser Permanente, Stockton, California.

Internet Resources
American Association of Retired People (AARP)
www.aarp.org/relationships/caregiving

www.caregiver.com
For caregivers, about caregivers, by caregivers

www.caregiving.com
"Helping you help family members and friends."

www.familycaregiving101.org
Place to find caregiving assistance.

www.medicinenet.com/caregiving/article.htm
Excellent site for information

National Alliance for Caregiving
4720 Montgomery Lane, 2nd Floor
Bethesda, MD 20814
www.naccaregiving.org

National Family Caregivers Association
http://www.familycaregiving.org
www.nfcacares.org

BIBLIOGRAPHY

Anema, Durlynn. *Late Life: Socialization and Concerns of Older Americans.* Lodi, California: DCAG Associates, 1989.

Beach, Shelly. *Precious Lord, Take My Hand: Meditations for Caregivers.* Grand Rapids, Michigan: Discovery House Publishers, 2007.

Berman, Claire. *Caring for Yourself While Caring for Your Aging Parents, 3rd Edition.* New York: Henry Holt and Company, 2005.

Coste, Joanne Koenig. *Learning to Speak Alzheimer's.* Boston/New York: Houghton Mifflin Company, 2003.

Henry, Stella Mora R. N. with Ann Conoery. *The Eldercare Handbook: Difficult Choices, Compassionate Solutions.* New York: HarperCollins Publishers, 2006.

Jacobs, Barry J., PsyD. *The Emotional Survival Guide for Caregivers.* New York: The Guilford Press, 2006.

Lynn, Dr. Dorree and Isaacs, Florence. *When the Man You Love Is Ill.* New York: Marlowe and Company, 2007.

Mace, Nancy L., M. A. and Rabins, Peter V., M. D. *The 36-Hour Day, 3rd Edition.* Baltimore: The John Hopkins University Press, 1999.

McLeod, Beth Witrogen. *Caregiving: The Spiritual Journey of Love, Loss and Renewal.* New York: John Wiley and Sons, Inc., 1999.

Samples, Pat; Larsen, Diane; Larsen, Marvin. *Self-Care for Caregivers: A Twelve Step Approach.* Center City, Minnesota: Hazelden Foundation, 1991.

Sheehy, Gail. *Passages in Caregiving: Turning Chaos into Confidence.* New York: William Morrow, 2010.

Thompson, Gretchen. *God Knows Caregiving Can Pull You Apart: 12 Ways to Keep It All Together.* Notre Dame, Indiana: Sorin Books, 2002.